AUTISM SPECTRUM DISORDER

A Guide for Educators and Parents

ANGELA A. EGBIKUADJE, MFT, MAOB, PhD.

DEDICATION

To all children with
Developmental and Intellectual Disabilities

CONTENTS

INTRODUCTION

The increasing number of individuals with autism spectrum disorder (ASD) in Nigeria is a major concern for many educators and parents, who continue to be faced with many challenges in finding the best resources to help children and adolescents with the disorder. Although researchers such as Bakare, Ebigbo, and Ubochi (2012) have speculated that the prevalence of autism spectrum disorder in sub-Saharan Africa is 0.7% higher than three decades ago, there are no clear statistics on the number of individuals with autism spectrum disorder in Nigeria. Notwithstanding the fact that the actual number of people impacted by ASD in Nigeria and throughout sub-Saharan Africa is not known, it is my hope that increased awareness of autism spectrum disorders in the different cities and the major villages in Nigeria will make more parents and caretakers willing to seek services for their children with symptoms of autism spectrum disorder. This book explains autism spectrum disorder in simple language to give all readers full understanding of the disorder. Although my goal is not to make the readers professionals in the diagnosis and treatment of ASD, I want all readers of this book to try to enlighten their friends and the community at large about the prevalence of autism spectrum disorders as well as the numerous ways that individuals impacted by ASD can be helped to live more independently. The major purpose of this book is to broaden the knowledge of parents and special education teachers in Nigeria concerning what autism spectrum disorder means and how people can assist children and adolescents with autism spectrum disorder to live goal- and purpose-driven lives.

For many years, parents and educators in Nigerian society have looked for ways to assist children manifesting symptoms of autism spectrum disorder. The complexities of behaviors seen in the symptoms presented by children with autism spectrum disorder make it difficult for many parents and educators to recognize the behaviors and mannerisms that are unique to ASD. Some Nigerians have mythical views of ASD. Some believe that a child with autistic qualities is a curse to a family, is possessed by an evil spirit, or is a special messenger from the evil world. The thinking that ASD equates to insanity is another major factor explaining why many children and adolescents diagnosed with ASD are not taken at an earlier age for appropriate services. Rather, once they become adolescents, they are allowed to roam the streets, and many times they become objects of mockery. Not surprisingly, Bakare and colleagues (2012) found that more than 50% of healthcare workers located in the southeast and the far south regions of Nigeria linked childhood autism with natural, preternatural, and supernatural causes. The authors further found that the more a healthcare worker was exposed to children diagnosed with ASD, the more likely that the healthcare worker was to believe the causes of the disorder was not supernatural. Therefore, this book was designed to help parents, educators, healthcare workers, and the general public understands the facts of ASD and learns how to assist children and adolescents with ASD.

Early intervention is paramount in enabling people with the disorder to live full lives. Intervention includes effective diagnosis and appropriate treatment strategies once the child begins to manifest symptoms of ASD. The symptoms of autism spectrum disorders must be reviewed in terms of the typical developmental milestones for the majority of the children. These early signs of autism spectrum disorders which will be discussed at length in subsequent chapters include the baby's inability to "babble" or inability to speak, difficulties smiling or expressing emotions when prompted by siblings or mother, poor eye contact, does not seem happy, difficulties with grasping objects or toys or might not like to play, and might appear to have a hearing problem. Early and appropriate interventional strategies enable the child with ASD to grow up with the skills that will allow them not only to become self-sufficient, but also to remain independent. Some individuals with mild ASD symptoms and no coexisting intellectual or mental health disorder can achieve university degrees if they are diagnosed early and provided with appropriate learning strategies beginning from a very young age. Helping the child with ASD learn is not the duty of the teacher alone, but the child's parents and the entire family.

In Nigeria, the presence of social stigma negatively impact individuals with autism spectrum disorder. Although social stigma appears to be a "silent" factor, it has caused many educated and non-educated parents to hide their children from the public. Children with autism spectrum disorders are sometimes locked up in their houses and isolated for fear of public scrutiny of the family. Sadder still is the fact that sometimes individuals with autism spectrum disorders are not allowed to socialize even with their siblings in the house. It is my wish that the information in this book will provide parents and family members of children with mild to severe symptoms of ASD to see the beauty in their children. I want all parents to know that having a child born with ASD is no fault of theirs and the child does not deserve to be punished. Every child has value, even those who appear to possess minimal talents and whose future does not seem bright.

A major goal of this book is to provide special education teachers information and skills that will enable them to explore ways to address the difficult behaviors exhibited by students with ASD. My interaction with special education teachers in Nigeria as well as parents has shown me that it is the problematic behaviors of students more than their learning problems that cause frustration. It is not unusual for parents to take their children to a psychiatrist and for teachers to encourage parents to take their children with ASD to a physician for psychiatric or psychotropic medications. Although it is not ethically wrong to medicate individuals with ASD, it is important for parents and educators to explore the various psychological interventions, psychosocial support, and behavioral strategies before seeking the help of a psychiatrist. Psychiatric medication is not the only answer to the difficult behavior problems that can be posed by children with ASD symptoms. Rather, many children and adolescents with ASD show significant improvement when behavior strategies are implemented with unconditional and genuine love. It is very important for parents and educators not to underestimate the degree of sensitivity experienced by individuals with ASD. To say the least, the children with ASD know who cares and truly loves them. In my years of experience as a therapist, I have seen children whose parents thought there was no hope for change in their behaviors turn around and become responsible.

Nonetheless, parents who insist on psychotropic or psychiatric medication for their children with ASD should first explore all the long-term side effects of these drugs as well as the long-term benefits. A question parents and teachers should ask before insisting that the child with ASD be prescribed medication is this: "Who is the medication going to benefit the most?" If the answer is the parent seeking respite time and relief, then reevaluate the decision. There might be better options such as employing a nanny or a caregiver. On the other hand, the parent or teacher might be seeking psychotropic medication for their child because the severity of the symptoms are injurious to the child or others; in cases of intense violence, uncontrollable aggression, and infliction of self-harm or harm to others, medications might be necessary.

The need to provide resources for the many Nigerian parents and educators cannot be overemphasized. Parents and educators must broaden their knowledge of what autism spectrum disorder is and entails and how they can contribute towards the ability of the child or adolescent with ASD to live a goal-oriented life. Even though understanding ASD and other developmental disabilities is not easy for parents or educators, believing that knowledge is power, being optimistic, and opening oneself to learn will be keys to improving the life of the child or adolescent with ASD.

A PERSONAL STORY

About 23 years ago, while I was on vacation from the university, I was assigned to a classroom of about 10 to 12 children with different types of developmental disabilities and medical conditions including Down syndrome, cerebral palsy, and maybe autism. The only instructions I was given was to try to teach the students the alphabet for a few minutes, teach them a few numbers, put on some music and let them sing along, let them do some art work, and at recess help those with walking difficulties go out onto the playground. One other staff was in the classroom to help me with the children.

To be honest, despite the instructions provided, I was lost. At that time, I had no knowledge of developmental disabilities and I was an undergraduate student in the field of accounting. I looked at all the children sitting in the classroom and began to feel sympathy for them. I went completely blank at one point during the day. I am not sure today what I did with them back then, but one thing I remember for sure: I was scared and confused trying to think of the best way to help them get through the day . . . and of how I was going to get through the day as well. For the entire day, my heart went out to each child in the classroom. My greatest confusion can be summed up in one question I could not answer: "How can any person teach these children?"

I am sure some special education teachers who have gone through the academic work of learning how to teach children with developmental disorders and are yet to have real classroom experience can relate to my experience. Is it not true that the theories learned in universities on how to impact knowledge sometimes don't translate to real-life experience where human conditions are more complex and behaviors are difficult to predict? This is the reason for this book. It is my hope that teachers will be encouraged and, most importantly, experience internal fulfillment as they attempt to assist children and adolescents with autism spectrum disorder live a better and a more fulfilled life.

Going back on my story as an inexperienced special education teacher 23 years ago, I recall one child in particular who stood out -- what a handsome young boy with serious physical disabilities yet quite talented in music. I wonder where he is now. I wish I knew back then what I know now! This young boy's experience would have been different if I had known how to diagnose developmental disabilities and how to develop effective learning strategies and plans for the developmentally disabled. This is not in any way to suggest that the services that were provided to the students at the time were completely ineffective. However, exploration of this young boy's skill for music might have helped him develop that ability further and could have been used as a yardstick to discover other talents the young boy might have had. To be more specific, a teacher knowledgeable in developmental disabilities would have explored what skills the child possessed in the area of spatial abilities and given him the tools to develop and enjoy those skills.

For parents and educators who might not understand what spatial abilities mean or why such knowledge is important in helping children, here is a simple definition: Spatial ability is "skill in representing, transforming, generating, and recalling symbolic, non-linguistic information" (Linn & Peterson, 1985, p. 1482). In other words, spatial ability is a type of intelligence that involves non-verbal communication such as skills in music and mathematical problem solving. As I look back and consider the musical talent of the young boy I encountered in the classroom many years ago, I realize that although he did not receive a formal diagnostic screening, his presentations and skills seem consistent at a certain level with those of some children diagnosed with ASD who excel in mathematics and other problem solving activities that don't involve use of expressive and written language. Diagnosticians help uncover the skills that are inherent in each unique child diagnosed with autism spectrum disorder.

In the past, fear, a sense of helplessness, and a somewhat desolate feeling that children with developmental disabilities are incapable of learning prevented me from exploring special education. I did not think that attempting to teach special-needs children was worth the effort; I needed to focus my energies on individuals who will change the world. You know what? I was wrong. And if any educator or parent has such thoughts, they are wrong too. Changing the world does not necessarily mean doing something on a large scale. Parents and educators can change the world - one child at a time.

Furthermore, after gaining extensive knowledge and experience with individuals diagnosed with autism spectrum disorders and other developmental disorders, I have a different perspective now on learning and how it relates to the individual born with a developmental disorder. It is my goal that as a result of reading this book, parents and educators will be more confident and have renewed strength that will allow them the freedom to explore different learning options for individuals diagnosed with autism spectrum disorder. Not to make the picture too rosy. . . . Although many children with mild symptoms of autism spectrum disorders are capable of learning and achieving high levels of education, a few are incapable of learning or can learn very little due to co-morbid disorders.

ORGANIZATION OF THE BOOK

This book is simple; it is divided into two parts. It is very important that parents and teachers learn about the different factors that can affect learning for the individual diagnosed with autism spectrum disorder. Thus, the first part of this book explores the different psychiatric and medical conditions that can impact learning for the child or adolescent with ASD. The focus in the first part of the book is helping educators and parents understand the differences between the various conditions that can influence learning for the child or adolescent with ASD. Several psychological disorders are described and discussed: what used to be diagnosed as mental retardation and is currently called intellectual disability, attention deficit hyperactivity disorder, oppositional defiant disorder and conduct disorder, depression, anxiety, schizophrenia, and unclassified psychotic disorder and mood disorder.

Furthermore, the first part of the book contains a brief examination of the impact of medical diagnoses such as Down syndrome, cerebral palsy, fragile X syndrome, seizures, and medical problems such as enuresis and encopresis. The ways these conditions affect the individual diagnosed with autism spectrum disorder are explained. The goal of this discussion is to inform parents about the existence of these disorders rather than to teach them how to diagnose them. It is my hope that by the end of the book, parents and educators will be able to recognize the presence of any of the above listed psychological or medical conditions and make appropriate referral to clinical psychologists or trained mental health diagnosticians when they suspect that one or more may co-exist with autism spectrum disorder in a particular child.

These conditions definitely have a significant impact on learning. The myth that the individual with ASD is not able to learn persists largely because some individuals with ASD experience learning difficulties because of other medical or psychological conditions. For the child with ASD with no co-morbid factors, learning is not as challenging. Even when teaching a child is extremely difficult, or it is seldom impossible, no child should be left behind in the learning process because each child, whether developmentally disabled or not, is unique and possesses talents that are useful either in the classroom or outside the classroom. Identifying their unique talents, no matter how irrelevant they might seem, brings joy to many families and to the individuals with autism spectrum disorder. Teachers and parents should never allow discouragement or frustrations to prevent them from helping children discover their unique abilities. Be grateful for the opportunity to bring joy where joy does not seem obvious.

To add a brief personal note. . . . When I was growing up, my father used to always say, "Nobody is dumb." As a child, I had difficulty understanding why a student who was failing all her classes was not "dumb." You know what? The fact is that the student was yet to recognize her strengths and weaknesses. Your report card does not always reflect who you are, what you are capable of, and what you will become in the future.

The second part of this book focuses on behavior strategies I have designed and implemented in my services to developmentally disabled individuals. Although the model I designed has not been empirically tested, it has worked well for my clients, in both Nigeria and the United States. It is a simple model and I believe it will be helpful to parents and educators working with persons with ASD who exhibit significant behavior problems.

Using this behavior model requires a thorough understanding of the precipitating factors that foster the problematic behaviors in individuals diagnosed with autism spectrum disorder. Without a definite and accurate diagnosis of the particular disorder an individual has, the behavior strategies might not work. For example, a very depressed child needs a great deal of attention because the depression or anxiety has to be alleviated before the child will comply with any behavior modification intervention. The goal of the behavior modification program is not to make the depressed child more depressed or the psychotic child more psychotic. It is to foster healing and, in the long term, help individuals with autism spectrum disorder appreciate themselves more and help their parents and their educators enjoy being with them.

My approach to formulating a behavior modification plan is that the plan is an attempt to make individuals with autism spectrum disorder change the way they view life and behavior. Thus, I emphasize the rewards of positive behaviors rather than the consequences that results from negative behaviors. Concentrating on the negative often causes people to become immune to negativity and the consequences that follow, eventually depriving parents and educators of appropriate ways to change the behaviors. When parents or educators lack appropriate ways of changing negative behaviors, they have lost control and power. The loss of control and power can be devastating, and parents or educators who have been in this situation will agree that it is not a good place to be with their child or their student. The techniques I offer in this book are meant to serve as guides that will help both parents and teachers bring positive change to the individuals with ASD in their lives.

1

AUTISM SPECTRUM DISORDER: FACTS AND HOPES

In the Nigerian culture, as in most African cultures, the birth of the child is an occasion of joy, laughter, and celebration. No parent dreams of having children who will not be able to speak, will not want to have friends, will not walk or use their hands normally, or will not be able to play with their brothers and sisters. In fact, majority of parents in African cultures have more than one child because they believe the children will be play-mates and companions for their brothers and sisters. Parents assume their children will grow up and be able to take care of themselves as well as their parents. Parents have huge dreams for their children. Don't most parents take a lot for granted af-ter a child is born? It is just normal to assume that all will be fine with the child. Children with autism spectrum disorder are often unable to fulfill the dreams and expectations of their parents because they are different from typically developing children. Although the differences vary considerably from child to child in specifics and severity, two basic characteristics are common to children with ASD:

1. Difficulty in social Interaction and communication
2. Repetitive patterns of behaviors, interests, and mannerisms

Consider the very typical case of Sunny:

CASE STUDY 1-1

Sunny is 5 years old and he is not like my other children. He is my third child and I have four children. Sunny has refused to speak even though I have taken him to see several speech therapists. Nobody can tell me why he will not talk. I took him to see the doctor and the doctor just told me, "Some children are slow. Give him time." When I watch him sometimes, he is talking to himself and when I ask him to talk to me, he will keep quiet. Sunny will not play with his brothers and sisters. He will fight if they take his toys. Sunny cannot sit still and cannot concentrate and the only time that Sunny will agree to sit down is when he has to eat his favorite food, which is beans and fried plantain. He forgets easily. For example, just asking Sunny to call his brother, even though he would go to his brother, he will not tell him anything. If I don't hold his hand when we are outside, he will run and start hugging other people. He smiles sometimes to himself and when I ask him why he is smiling; he will just be looking at me. Tip toeing is his way of walking. I recently took Sunny to see the doctor again and he said that Sunny has no medical problem... What is happening to my child? I am so confused.

Although not all children with ASD fit the profile of Sunny, his story illustrates the importance of understanding the child's behaviors. The complexities of human behavior make it difficult for many parents to figure out the reasons behind their children's unique behaviors and mannerisms. A clear understanding of the problematic behaviors in children requires some knowledge of child development and what behaviors are typical at the different stages. Children will not necessarily meet their developmental milestones (walking, talking, etc.) at the same time, but ranges of typical times have been dictated from observation of biological and psychological phenomena. Now let us look at some of the major characteristics of Sunny that are causing her mother significant fears.

Communication. Effective communication enables parents to interact with their children and helps children get their needs met from a very young age. Therefore, we cannot overemphasize the importance of understanding the components of communication and its significance in human development from birth to adulthood. Generally, children begin to make meaningless but speech-like sounds at age 2 to 3 months, they begin to babble from 5 months, and they usually say their first word between the ages of 10 to 14 months (Feldman, 2003). Prior to age 2-3 months, however, infants are able to communicate with their mothers especially with the help of the sense of smell. According to Feldman, infants begin to hear prenatally and they are able to distinguish their mother from other women based on the sense of smell from ages 12 to 18 days. Sunny's mother's observations indicate that Sunny is having some problems with communication. Both expressive (spoken) language and receptive language (reactions to spoken language) are important areas of development for any child.

Social interaction. In Nigerian society, parents and educators sometimes underestimate the importance of appropriate social interaction skills. At first, children who do not engage in a lot of play activities from the start of their development are often seen as well behaved. In time, however, if children are not making friends, parents become concerned and may seek the help of doctors or teachers. When, as in the case of Sunny, the absence of friends occurs in conjunction with a myriad of other problems, there is cause for alarm. Social interaction is significant to a child's psychological health. Structural family therapists have shown that the social interaction and play that takes place between parents and children brings pleasure to the children and reduces tension in parent-child relationships (Minuchin, 1974).

On the other hand, when social interaction is excessive and makes the child increasingly restless, parents have reason for concern. In the case study, Sunny runs to strangers to hug them during social events or activities. This is unusual. In healthy social interactions, a person is involved in an activity with one or more other persons. Social interaction does not occur if one of the parties does not respond to the first party's invitation to play, or interact; the response is what is referred to as social reciprocity. Psychologically, reciprocal social interaction is very significant to a child's health, and such social interactions begin during infancy. For example, infants reciprocate smiles when they smile back during play. Reciprocal social interaction is "a process in which [a child's] behaviors invite further responses from parents and other caregivers, which in turn bring about further responses from the [child]" (Feldman, 2003, p. 201). Going back to the case study, it is evident that Sunny does not reciprocate in play. Sunny's mother seemed most concerned because Sunny's social interaction skills are not comparable with those of other children of the same age. Because Sunny has not been diagnosed with any medical condition, it is the role of the clinical psychologist to observe him, perhaps administer more tests, and determine how to best help Sunny.

Abnormal behaviors. Sunny's mother reported that Sunny talks and smiles to himself, he walks on tip toe instead of walking like other children of the same age, and he looks at her instead of responding with words. These behaviors are examples of abnormal behaviors frequently exhibited by children with ASD. Generally, parents, educators, and other people who have observed the children closely observe some abnormal or odd behaviors. Some commonly reported behaviors are washing the same dinner plate for over 10 minutes, banging on a table in a very rhythmic way, turning on and switching off lights, and rearranging objects or pictures in a particular manner. It is amazing to watch children with ASD run into their houses and see that the first thing they do is change the patterns of items on the floor or on a table. They know when the arrangement of such objects is changed, even if they have not seen them for 6 months.

RELEVANT DEVELOPMENTAL MILESTONES AND FINE MOTOR SKILL DEVELOPMENT

If parents and educators are to be able to detect behaviors that are not typical, they must be well versed in the norms of typical developmental milestones for children. Although Sunny's mother should be commended for making the effort to find out if her son has a medical condition, she is confused because she is unable to obtain answers about her son's delays and other problems. It is not unusual for parents such as Sunny's mother to resort to prayer and fasting or seek the help of traditional herbalists, but they would be less confused if they knew the milestones that are part of children's normal development and the ages at which they are usually achieved. So let us examine some of them in Table 1.

Table 1. Children's Motor Development Milestones

AGE (MONTHS)	MILESTONES AND MOTOR SKILL DEVELOPMENT
2-3	Ability to babble and make meaningless sounds
3 – 3½	Ability to roll over and spread hands apart
3.3 - 3½	Ability to grasp toys (rattles)
5-6	Ability to sit without support
7-7½	Ability to stand while holding onto an object such as a chair, a table, or humans
8-8½	Ability to grasp objects with thumb and fingers
10-14	Make up their first words.
11-11½	Ability to hold toys such as crayons and stand without support
11½ - 12½	Ability to walk and expected to walk well by 12½ months
14-16	Ability to play with bigger objects and toys. A time to watch because they pick up little marbles or stones from the floor and bring them to their mouths
24	Can imitate strokes on paper, can take a cup and bring it to their lips, can take a drink without spilling
33	Can copy circles and can actually learn

Note. Adapted from *Development across the Life Span* by R. S. Feldman, 2003, New York: Prentice Hall.

From the information in Table 1, three major areas of concerns are evident in the case study:

1. Speech – the ability to communicate verbally
2. Fine motor skills – the ability to use muscles in the fingers, lips, tongues, and toes in grasping
3. Overall learning ability – the ability to follow instructions

Sunny appears to be experiencing difficulties with speech and probably also with following directions. He seems to be able to feed himself and he can hold his toys and use them for play. The inability of children with ASD to complete tasks others of their age can do, to conveniently learn, or to engage in appropriate play continues to be major areas of concern for both parents and educators. Considering the range of autism spectrum disorders, there are variations in behaviors and the severity of the symptoms differs for each child. Some individuals have significant difficulties with their fine motor skills but they might have minimal difficulties with social/communication skills. The key to helping children is effective diagnosis and following through with effective interventions and strategies from an early age.

PHYSICAL MANIFESTATIONS AND AUTISM SPECTRUM DISORDER

The distinctive physical appearance and the motor mannerisms of children with ASD cause some people to label these children "different." Many psychologists make an initial diagnosis of ASD from a child's physical manifestations and motor mannerisms. In Nigerian society, the physical manifestations of the child with ASD sometimes cause people to walk away from the child or look more closely to determine what is different about the child. Physical manifestations such as not being able to hold a small ball, tiptoeing, walking in front of moving traffic, running to embrace a stranger, or gazing intently at an object create embarrassment in parents, and they may feel shame. It is the shame that parents feel that triggers their desire to hide their children from their peers or the children's peers. Nigerian parents highly value physical attractiveness of children; therefore most parents of children with ASD who exhibit obvious physical symptoms and mannerisms are often ashamed to be seen with their children in public in Nigeria.

Nonetheless, hiding children or preventing the child with serious and obvious physical mannerisms and symptoms from participating in family events do not resolve any problems. I encourage parents and caregivers to seek the necessary help very early in the life of the child. Assistance starts with identifying experts in the field of mental health, having them conduct a thorough psychological assessment, and locating schools that have teachers who can effectively teach children with ASD.

Diagnostic guides such as the Diagnostic Manual for Mental Disorders have established the fact that the difficulties children with ASD experience in social interactions can be reduced over time with effective interventions and with parents' direct involvement in the child's treatment. Whether the physical manifestations of ASD in children can be changed over time has not been scientifically proven. Therapists expect, however, that psychological intervention and physical therapy sessions beginning early in the lives of children with ASD should bring some improvement in their fine motor abilities. As long as the children do not have other severe motor difficulties, they can be expected to learn how to mask their problems as they grow into adulthood. For example, the 19- year old male with ASD who knows that he cannot keep his fingers steady when he is holding a remote control will find ways to avoid holding or using a remote control in a public place.

SAMENESS AND AUTISM SPECTRUM DISORDER

Parents and educators continue to wonder why the child with ASD prefers routine or going through every day in the same way. Insistence on doing the same thing every time, every hour, and every day is one of the characteristic of the disorder. No doubt many parents and educators have found the sameness characteristic of the child with ASD frustrating. Common examples are insisting on watching a specific television program or insisting that only a particular piece of music be played irrespective of the time of day. The child might also refuse certain food in the morning and not in the afternoon. Although for the most part, parents are able to redirect children with ASD to be cognizant of the needs of others, the task of parenting a child with ASD is undoubtedly challenging. Instructing and redirecting the child several times during the day can be exhausting. From a positive perspective, the child's need for sameness can minimize some of the other symptoms frequently exhibited by the child with ASD. Creating a structured environment for the child minimizes some of the problems that come with the need for sameness. Effective design of the daily structure of events reinforces the symptom of sameness. Without being aware of what is happening, the children can be guided by the structured environment to adhere to routines created by their parents, caregivers, or teachers. The adults can change the environment, and thus the children's behaviors, without the children being conscious of the changes. In this way parents and educators are able to use the "sameness skills" of the children to their advantage as well as to the benefit of the children. The child is deprived of neither comfort nor the basic essentials when structures are appropriately created and used.

FEARS AND TREATMENT

Understandably, parents face fears when they discover and come to terms with the fact that their child is different. Although parents in Nigeria, especially mothers, might notice that their children are exhibiting some problematic symptoms before they are 1 year old, they do not seek treatment until they find out that the child is not meeting developmental milestones in a timely manner. When children do not speak and do not respond to verbal commands, parents worry and they often seek help. Nigerian parents seek help from medical experts or from traditional (native) doctors. However, once they begin to suspect that their child has significant developmental problems; their fears frequently hinder them from pursuing other treatment options. They are often ashamed and ignorance keeps them from talking about the symptoms exhibited by their child. What is most ignored by parents and least explored at the initial stages of the child's development is the possibility of developmental disability.

When parents come to terms with their child's developmental problems their first question is commonly "What is happening to my child?" Sometimes parents ask, "What have I done wrong? Who did this to me?" The amount of time many parents spend questioning why their children are not meeting their developmental milestones appropriately is excessive, and it is detrimental to the children who need help and services starting from a young age. It is normal for parents to go through a grieving process that includes questioning, but they need to focus on solutions. They need to move forward with finding the best services for their children. Excessive questionings and playing the blame game only creates difficulties for the child and the parents. Questioning and blaming give room for irrelevant thoughts and can be quite emotionally draining.

The more time spent wailing and wishing things were different; the less time is available for children with autism spectrum disorder to discover who they truly are and what they can achieve.

PARENTS' STANCE AND EARLY SIGNS OF AUTISM SPECTRUM DISORDER IN NIGERIA

The reason developmental disabilities such as autism spectrum disorders are not diagnosed early in Nigeria or suspected by parents is the strong belief that "that sort of thing cannot happen to me." Or, as the expression in Nigeria goes, "It is not my portion." Because knowledge about autism spectrum disorders is limited and the manner in which children exhibit symptoms is confusing, parents sometimes suspect witchcraft, curses, or other demonic influences account for their children's behaviors. Although no parent wishes to have a child born with ASD, when parents do have a child with ASD it is important that they realize that their child is human, has capabilities, and deserves their love.

It is also important that they recognize the condition as early as possible. I have heard parents state time and again, "My child was normal. He just could not speak . . . or spoke a little. . . . And then all these other things started happening. . . Now he cannot feed himself." Many parents report that delay in speech or verbal language was the sign that caused them to explore the idea that their child might have a developmental problem. Some mothers attribute their child's developmental problems to the depression and sadness they felt during pregnancy; other parents decide to seek help from medical professionals because at some time they concluded that their child was deaf. Some parents say their child cries most of the time and dislikes play that other children of similar age enjoy, but they don't know why. Nigerian parents obviously have difficulty understanding and dealing with the many facets of ASD.

Parents' anxiety could be lowered and their children diagnosed earlier if they knew more about ASD, particularly from the perspectives of other parents. Mothers and fathers of children with ASD need to share their stories to provide insight and support to parents in similar situations. If parents such as the mother of Sunny were to talk about their pregnancies, their children's birth, and the onset of the symptoms in their children, other parents would feel less isolated and have greater hope for their families. A team of parents can do more for their children than one set of parents alone. As more parents and educators in Nigeria gain greater understanding of autism spectrum disorder, they might spread the information to their neighbors, friends, and the public at large. The spread of knowledge is the beginning of the delivery of better services.

The improvement of learning outcomes for students with ASD is a priority among parents, and early diagnosis and treatment interventions permit more to be achieved in this area. To improve learning outcomes for these students in the Nigerian culture, educators and school administrators must be trained to understand what strategies are effective. Attempts to implement interventions and introduce new teaching techniques for children with ASD will be ineffective without proper understanding of the children and their environment. Consequently, parents, educators, and school administrators must embrace education about the social, psychological, physical, spiritual, and family environment of children with ASD.

I have a few words of encouragement for parents who are asking the same question as Sunny's mother: "What is wrong with my child?" The child with ASD characteristics was not born that way because of anything you did that was wrong. The child born with ASD will learn more words than you think. The child born with ASD will develop more independent living skills than you can imagine. All that is required is that you teach that child with love.

OTHER CONDITIONS THAT MIGHT OCCUR WITH AUTISM SPECTRUM DISORDER

There are several conditions that sometimes co-exist with ASD. Some are medical conditions, some are mental health conditions, and some are learning problems. A few of the common ones are:

1. Intellectual disabilities
2. Rett's disorder
3. Attention deficit hyperactivity disorder
4. Oppositional defiant disorder
5. Affective disorders such anxiety and depression
6. Psychotic disorders such as schizophrenia

Intellectual disabilities. Intellectual disabilities impact learning for the child, adolescent, or adult with ASD. Information on learning disabilities is explored in chapter 2.

Rett's disorder. There is ongoing controversy amongst experts in the field of mental health regarding the classification of Rett's disorder as an autism spectrum disorder. Whatever the official classification, children diagnosed with Rett's disorder most times show the same symptoms as those diagnosed with ASD. According to the *Diagnostic and Statistical Manual for Mental Health* (American Psychiatric Association, 2000), children diagnosed with Rett's disorder have difficulties with speech, problems with the use of their hands, and poor fine motor skills. They are prone to seizures and some have profound mental impairment. Rett's disorder is more common among females than males.

CAUSE OF AUTISM

Autism spectrum disorder is not mental retardation nor is it due to mental retardation. What does cause the condition? Researchers have not found a definitive answer. The increased association of different medical and mental health conditions with autism spectrum disorder has led some to suggest that these conditions have some causal link to ASD, but no such link has been found. Some researchers believe that identifying the cause would at least point toward a cure. All that we know at this time is that there are no scientific explanations, no facts, and no proven links that tell us the exact cause or causes of autism spectrum disorder.

2

LEARNING

In Nigeria, the way parents, educators, and the public at large look at learning and education for students with special needs is to evaluate the roles of the special education teacher, the government, and the education board in creating and promoting an effective learning environment for students. For the child with autism spectrum disorder, as for all children, learning begins at home and continues to be fostered in the home. As soon as ASD is suspected, learning interventions should commence in order for the child to have a positive learning outcome (Strain, Schwartz, & Barton, 2011). Involvement in recreational and other social activities is critical to the learning that is provided for children with ASD because they have deficiencies in social interaction and social reciprocity. The parents of children with ASD, not their caregivers or their siblings, are their first teachers. Second to the parents are trained special educators and then leaders of the community and church groups to which they belong. Therefore parents need to understand the significance of psychological testing for the developmentally delayed; accurate diagnosis at a young age is essential for implementing good teaching strategies and realizing optimum learning outcomes.

For many years, there have been ongoing controversies about the extent of academic achievement a child with a diagnosis of autism spectrum disorder can achieve. Within the Nigerian population, there are no data to indicate whether children diagnosed with ASD have attained more than secondary school education. However, my discussions with some special education teachers and my review of an article by Josephine Igbinovia (2012) have made clear to me that some children in Nigeria with ASD are graduating from secondary schools. That fact suggests that the number of children diagnosed with autism spectrum disorder enrolling in vocational schools is rising, and teachers and school administrators at the secondary level and higher need to be current in the learning strategies that enable individuals with ASD to succeed in school and improve their lives. Whether students with autism spectrum disorder graduate from secondary school or learn a vocational trade, parents and educators must not relent in their efforts to assist them in recognizing their talents and skills while they are young and teachable. These efforts require that parents and teachers understand the kinds of teaching methodologies that are effective with students diagnosed with autism spectrum disorder; unrealistic expectations from parents or educators have been found to be very detrimental not only to the physical and psychological health of the child with ASD, but also to their overall view of life.

IMPACT OF LEARNING ON THE CHILD WITH ASD

The degree of severity of the child's ASD symptoms determines the extent of learning the child will be able to attain. Children with very mild symptoms are able to attend regular schools and are capable of competing with their peers in those schools. Even though they are able to compete with students in regular school, it is very important that parents and educators individualize the education plan for students with ASD and help them to recognize their talents and skills.

Furthermore, the ability of children with ASD to learn depends to a large extent on their unique talents as well as on a number of variables including parents' interest in their child's learning experience, parents' economic status, and a positive social environment. Another variable affecting ability to learn is the presence of medical or mental health problems. For example, a few of the mental and medical problems that influence learning are intellectual disability, attention deficit hyperactivity disorder, oppositional defiant disorder, schizophrenia, depression, anxiety, and gastroenteritis. These conditions make learning difficult.

Sometimes, educators hold controversial beliefs that hinder children's learning. The common perception that teaching a child with a developmental disability is a waste of time has an obvious negative impact on teaching. When educators do not believe their teaching will have an effect, they are not likely to deliver the best instruction and their students with ASD are shortchanged. Many teachers in the field of special education have a passion for their special job and approach it with enthusiasm and optimism for each child in their classroom. Their confident attitude and belief that their students can learn are likely to have a positive impact on their students' learning.

LEARNING AND THE SOCIAL ENVIRONMENT

Children with autism spectrum disorder are limited in their ability to participate appropriately in their social environment (Strain et al., 2011). However, researchers have shown correlation between learning for ASD students and their social environment (Estes, Rivera, Bryan, & Dawson, 2011; Kuhlthau et al., 2010). Social skills deficits—specifically, difficulties with communication, problems with fine motor manipulation, obsessive (repetitive) behavior patterns, and stereotypically odd patterns of behavior—negatively impact learning for students with ASD. Although the extent of the relationship between learning and problems in social interaction varies from one individual to another, Jones and colleagues (2009) demonstrated that adolescents with ASD can reach high levels of achievement in academic subjects. The researchers found that approximately 72.7% of 14- to 16-year-old students with ASD in their study were skilled in at least one academic subject such as in reading, spelling, comprehension, arithmetic, and broader mathematic skills. They encouraged parents and educators to be vigilant in their children's education so that the academic skills and talents of their children with ASD don't go unnoticed.

Two strategies that have been found to be productive for students with ASD is to teach them in their natural environment and to focus teaching on helping them develop better and more positive interaction skills (Strain et al., 2011). Teachers, parents, and caregivers of children with ASD need to encourage formal learning from an early age in order to help the children become familiar with the learning environment. Familiarity with the social environment in which education takes place is very important to the ability of the child with ASD to learn, and the earlier the child is introduced to the specific environment, the greater the familiarity can grow. Estes et al. (2011) noted that early intervention seems to reduce the negative impact of the social environment; they found that a large number of children with ASD improved significantly in their intellectual abilities as well as behavioral functioning due to early interventions.

A word of caution is in order, especially for parents and educators in Nigeria. Unfortunately, rejection of children with ASD is not uncommon, and parents and educators must be cognizant of any experience of rejection that children with ASD experience in their social environment. The odd mannerisms that children with ASD exhibit tend to make them objects of mockery and victims of bullies in primary and secondary schools in Nigeria.

ACADEMIC PERFORMANCE
AND INTELLIGENCE

Intellectual abilities are usually defined separately from academic achievements. Many of the great scholars, who study intelligence, including Binet, Wechsler, Gardner, Sattler, and Freeman, define intelligence in terms of the manner in which individuals react to their environment. In other words, adaptation and problem solving skills are part of intelligence. In essence, these authors view intelligence not only in terms of an individual's cognitive functioning, but also in terms of how the individual reacts to the demands of the environment, which might require what we refer to in Nigeria as "the not so common sense." On the other hand, academic achievement or performance has been defined strictly in terms of individuals' ability to do well in the skills taught to them. The skills may have been taught in classes in a formal school system or they may have been learned from parents or other caregivers. Academic achievement is usually measured by evaluating performance of the skills that children learn through direct observation or observations from their instructors (Sattler, 2001).

Intelligence should not be confused with academic performance. When assessment of intelligence is based on measures of academic performance, the potential of the child is crippled. The confusion of intelligence and performance is detrimental to the self-esteem of any child. It permits skills that are potentially ingenious to go unnoticed or unappreciated.

Intelligence is much more than academic performance. In Nigeria, parents and the general public use academic performance as a major yardstick to measure the future of a child. I sincerely hope that by the end of this chapter, parents and educators will begin to view the future of any child with ASD from the perspective of the psychological definition of intelligence rather than based on how the student performs in the classroom environment. This perspective means that students with ASD can demonstrate intelligence and learning as they perform daily independent living tasks such as walking, bathing or showering, eating, washing their clothing, and accomplishing other hygiene tasks.

The intelligence of the child with ASD can also be measured by their ability to express their needs using appropriate and culturally acceptable language. Although children with severe symptoms might be totally dependent on their parents or caregivers for their daily living tasks throughout their lives, let us not ignore the many children with ASD who will excel in tasks that require general intelligence and limited academic performance.

In the large view of a child's capacity to succeed, intelligence is a single phenomenon that cannot be divided into separate compartments. Sattler (2001) described intelligence as operating within the framework of multiple factors including reasoning, memory, adaptive functioning, problem solving, mental speed and creativity, linguistic proficiency, sensory perception, general knowledge of the environment, and goal setting. Intelligence encompasses the entire abilities of all the human faculties: the mind, the hands and feet, and all the senses. Obviously, then, the child with ASD, who may be impaired in some faculties and not in others, has intelligence and therefore has the ability to learn.

As a clinical psychologist who helps children with disabilities exhibit positive behaviors, I know that intelligence has a behavioral component. Behaviors are functions of the activities of the intellect. Yes! Some may think that negative behaviors result from lack of rationalization, but the fact is that every behavior, whether it is spontaneous, impulsive, or deliberate, results from some activity of the intellect. The intensity of the activities of the human mind in different people is the bone of contention.

Just as behavior is a function of the intellect, so also is the intellect stimulated by behaviors. Consequently, training children and adolescents with ASD to develop the behaviors that constitute positive life skills sharpens their intelligence. Teaching survival tactics, practicing basic daily living activities, and providing vocational training is necessary educational strategies. Teachers need to address both intelligence and academic achievement of students with ASD to help them improve the quality of their lives.

COMMUNICATION AND AUTISM SPECTRUM DISORDER

Effective communication, which is the ability of an individual to interact with others through the use of words or gestures, is one of the best tools for assessing the responsiveness of individuals to what they are taught. Jones and colleagues (2009) identified primary social and communication difficulties as obvious explanations for the difficult classroom behaviors exhibited by some children with ASD. They recommended that teachers give particular attention to those students who have severe autism spectrum disorder symptoms so they can address any coexisting disabilities during the learning process. Teachers give students with ASD the greatest benefit when they identify and build on the strengths of the students, increasing their potential for success. This is especially true for students with strengths in mathematics, science, or other academic subjects.

The inability of children with ASD in Nigeria to engage effectively in social interaction with their parents, teachers, and peers through effective communication is a great concern. Communication between children with ASD and their parents, their siblings, and their caregivers is so important because it fosters learning for them and it also validates their efforts to improve in their learning. In a study of the quality of family life for children with varied intellectual disabilities in Nigeria, Ajuwon and Brown (2012) found that "meaningful communication" between children with intellectual disabilities and their parents was associated with improved learning in the children.

EFFECTIVE STRATEGIES FOR IMPROVING SOCIAL COMMUNICATION SKILLS IN CHILDREN WITH ASD

Simple alphabet and word learning. As the child with ASD attempts to communicate a specific need or desire through gestures or other forms of body language and the child's parents are able to identify the need the child expresses, the parents write the need the child is depicting on a piece of paper. The parents show the written word to the child and read the word aloud. They encourage the child to say the word aloud. For example, a boy who is hungry walks to his mother, who is sitting in the living room, then goes to the refrigerator and opens and closes the door of the refrigerator, then returns to his mother, and stands and stares at her, hoping she understands his desire. The mother writes the word "hungry" and prods her son to say "hungry." When the child says the word, the mother gives him something to eat. Although this exercise may sound tedious, it usually takes fewer than 5 minutes to get the child to actually repeat the word. After the exercise, the mother displays the paper with the word on it in a position where the child can see it throughout the day. It is parents' responsibility to encourage their children with ASD to speak to them.

Imitation. When children are very young, talking toys fascinate them. If children with ASD have talking or singing toys, they can be encouraged to repeat what they hear the toys say. Imitation is an effective strategy for improving communication in children with ASD (Strain et al., 2012; Young et al., 2011). Imitation is similar to structured play. When talking or singing toys are unavailable, parents and teachers can mimic such toys as they play with their children. Basically, parents and educators need to encourage the child with ASD to find speaking fun even though the words might be slurred or inaudible as first. Practice is the key. Do not be afraid to explore the child's skills. Many children with ASD can interact fairly well through gestures, but parents should not get too comfortable with that form of communication simply because they are able to understand their child's gestures or mannerisms. Instead they should be creative in finding fun ways to encourage the child with ASD to imitate specific functional words—words they will need in everyday social interactions.

Fun and laughter. Laughter, fun, and smiles are encouraging for the child with ASD. Some children may want to play all the time, and having fun together is a good way to get their attention and trust. Once that attention and trust is understood as love, the child will surprise you with some verbal remarks. A very good play activity for children with ASD is taking a favorite toy, hiding it from their sight, and asking them to look for it around you. When the children are unable to locate the toy, you produce it suddenly and show it to them. It is very important that the children do not get distracted during the play and get caught up with other activities. If that occurs, your play has gotten boring for the children and it will not be productive.

You can have fun and laugh with your child in many different ways. Laughter and smiles nearly always make the child with ASD feel accepted. I have found play very beneficial in improving learning for children with ASD. Parents should never stop playing with their children. Use play to teaching one word to your child every day, perhaps encouraging them to say "thank you."

Children with ASD need to be taught communication skills that are useful in social settings, but the skills are taught most effectively in a non-threatening environment. Children with ASD generally prefer isolative play—playing by themselves—but they need to be able to interact appropriately with others. So teachers should organize peer-to-peer interaction programs in their classrooms. Peer-to-peer programs in the school environment must include supervised play activities that the child with ASD can tolerate. The play must be supervised so one child does not monopolize the toys or other objects used in the activity. Unsupervised play creates chaos in the classroom.

BOUNDARIES AND LEARNING

It is up to parents to teach their children with ASD from a young age the importance of maintaining effective boundaries. They need to know that embracing a stranger is not appropriate, that turning off lights when they have not been asked to do so is not acceptable, and that it is not permissible for them to walk into the teacher's office without knocking. Individuals with ASD will need to be continually educated on the importance of boundaries. They also need to learn to recognize who they are and to what extent others are allowed to be in close physical proximity to them. Discussion of boundaries is especially important as children approach puberty. Adolescents with ASD are just as confused and just as emotional as other preteens and teenagers.

PHYSICAL CHARACTERISTICS AND LEARNING

Fine motor difficulties. The extent of the fine motor difficulties the child with ASD experiences will determine the type of intervention the child needs. Physical therapy is most beneficial when it is begun very early in the life of the child. Children can improve in skills such as grasping if physical therapy is begun on time.

Repetitive (stereotypical) but odd behaviors. Children with moderate to severe symptoms of the disorder might exhibit serious problems with behaviors characterized as obsessions. An obsession might be finger flipping, rocking back and forth, fixing a gaze on another individual, or banging on a desk. Depending on the severity of this symptom, the parent or educator might either refer the child to a psychologist or try to redirect the child. Often it is the exhibition of odd, repetitive, and stereotypical behaviors that causes parents to seek the help of a psychiatrist for their child. Evaluate the intensity of the disturbing behavior before resorting to medications.

SELF-ESTEEM AND LEARNING

Children need to have decent self-esteem for learning to proceed effectively. Some children with ASD have incredible skills but their low self-esteem makes them feel ashamed and they keep their abilities to themselves. Praising and affirming the child, even for very minute achievements, is quite important in raising feelings of self-worth. Children with moderate to severe symptoms are aware that they are different from others. Let us not make them feel too different by limiting their potential by believing the myth that they are incapable of learning. Children with mild symptoms of the disorder might show low motivation for learning if they are not validated and provided the necessary help.

FOSTERING INTELLIGENCE, SOCIAL RECOGNITION, AND THE MEDIA

Building knowledge and skills is a process of moving from the known to the unknown. Improving learning for children with ASD has to take into consideration what the children know and like as well as what the parent or teacher want them to learn. A girl who is fascinated with a particular radio station's music or advertising jingle may resist learning something new if not allowed to repeat the music or advertisement. By all means, allow the girl to sing the song that is so significant to her and then you can begin teaching what is scheduled for the day. A classic example is trying to teach a boy with severe fine motor difficulties how to draw. Please: the child with such problem can't draw. However, if he has had sufficient physical therapy so that his fine motor skills have improved, by all means, let him draw whatever he can and praise him for the drawing notwithstanding the absence of neatness or accuracy. The experience of using the hand and fingers is more important than the outcome of the drawing on the paper. A child with severe motor skills problems, specifically intense difficulties with grasping, might be able to learn to develop better skills by watching a video clip of someone drawing an object. Or the child might be trained to communicate through music and dancing instead of drawing. For educators new to the field of special education: be brave and do not be discouraged from becoming creative and trying new things in teaching your lessons.

INDEPENDENT LIVING SKILLS AND LEARNING

The myth that individuals with autism spectrum disorder will not be able to care for themselves has continued to be proven wrong. As already mentioned, the ability of children or adolescents to develop basic independent living skills such as cooking, bathing themselves, doing their own laundry or washing their clothing, and practicing appropriate toileting and hygiene depend on several factors. Most importantly, their ability to develop independent living skills depends on the severity of their ASD symptoms. For some children and adolescents, especially those diagnosed with other disorders such as depression, serious medical problems, and/or physical disabilities, independent living skills are huge tasks and they are very slow to acquire each of these skills. For others, developing independent living skills comes more easily. Nonetheless, children and adolescents with ASD need to be assisted and carefully supervised until they are able to complete all the necessary tasks independently. Please teach them how to do these tasks rather than concluding that they are incapable of caring for themselves. Also refrain from giving children or adolescents with ASD verbal instructions and sending them off on their own to perform these independent living tasks without being there to help them. They need your loving presence.

LEARNING BY ASSOCIATION

Many children with ASD in Nigeria might be able to learn to perform their independent living tasks by making associations with items or activities they enjoy. For example, children who love music but do not like to shower might be encouraged to shower when their favorite music is turned on. The special education teacher can experiment with learning by association with individual students. Learning by association is based on the recognition that the teacher must get the attention of students before attempting to teach them. Parents and educators have to listen to children with ASD to discover their likes and dislikes. Using the "likes," which are the children's strengths, is what makes learning by association effective. Using the learning by association method brings out the child's giftedness or exceptional talents; it forces the educator to identify them and encourages the child to build on them. Again, go from the known to the known. Moving from the known to the unknown is a great teaching strategy.

ADAPTIVE FUNCTIONING AND LEARNING

How well individuals with ASD solve basic living problems, exercising adaptive functioning skills, depends mostly on their level of confidence in the environment in which they reside. Basic living problems include dealing with conflicts with or without help from others. Other basic living problems are obtaining food when no one is able to bring it to them and responding to a fight or a fire outbreak. Adaptive functioning is the ability to respond to changes in the environment and changes in daily routines. Adapting to daily routines might involve going to school each day, knowing what day of the week it is, and knowing the routine of each day. You might be surprised to know that some children with ASD who are unable to tell you what day of the week it is can tell you their daily routine for the day, such as going to church on a Sunday. Responsiveness to daily routines might involve developing goals for the day. A teacher or parent may help the child with ASD develop concrete goals such as taking a bath at a certain time in the evening. The child with ASD will become more skilled in setting goals, and thus at problem solving, if the goals are uncomplicated and easily understood. Children's overall ability to adapt to both familiar and unfamiliar environments and changing situations depend greatly on the survival skills they are taught and is also affected by their self- esteem and their specific disability.

THE INTEGRATIVE LEARNING APPROACH

In summary, learning for the individual with autism spectrum disorder requires an integrative approach and it must commence early, as soon as the disorder is suspected or professionally diagnosed. Ideally, the integrative learning approach for the child with ASD incorporates the expertise of these professionals: the school administrator, the teachers and teachers' assistants, the parents or guardians, the psychiatrist, the primary physician, the clinical psychologist, the speech therapist, the physical therapist, and the behavior specialist. In Nigeria, the different professionals who should be involved in improving learning for the child with ASD might not be readily available. It is most important, therefore, that parents and educators make every effort to involve as many of the professionals who are available and who will contribute positively to the learning process of the child with ASD. Furthermore, for the child with ASD academic learning is not as important as developing abilities for accomplishing life tasks. Thus their education should not be limited to what they are taught in school (academic subjects), but must also include what they learn over time in their functional environment (intellectual abilities). Finally, learning for the child or adolescent with ASD must be comprehensive enough to embrace all aspects of their lives. Yes, the teacher in the school has a huge role to play in facilitating the learning process for the child or adolescent with ASD, but so also does the parent, who has the responsibility of beginning the child on the path of learning.

3

AWARENESS AND THE MIND AND BODY

The underlying principle that guides awareness of the mind and the body is the ability of humans to remain attentive to themselves and their environment. For children with ASD, mind and body awareness includes the expectation that the children are able to recognize and communicate their needs and their desires to their parents or educators. At the same time, we expect children with ASD to be able to recognize the needs of those who are in their environment. Recognizing one's own needs as well as the needs of others is important because it is a step in improving one's life and achieving one's goals. Isn't the basis of daily human functioning the attempts to meet one's needs and the needs of others, be they the need to rest, to make money, to be popular, to stay healthy, or to be successful? Whatever needs are present, attentiveness to self and the environment are necessary to having those needs met. Children with ASD frequently have difficulty integrating their own thoughts and feelings while remaining sensitive to the needs of others (peers, parents, siblings, etc.).

INATTENTIVENESS, HYPERACTIVITY, AND DISTRACTIBILITY

The number of children with ASD and a co-morbid diagnosis of attention deficit hyperactivity disorder (ADHD) are increasing and have remained high (Adewuya & Famuyiwa, 2007; Gjevik, Eldevik, Fjaeran-Granum, & Sponheim, 2011). Inattentiveness and hyperactivity are major indicators of ADHD (Adewuya & Famuyiwa). No wonder children with ASD have difficulty emulating and developing appropriate social interaction skills! Although more scientific research measuring the awareness levels of children or adolescents with ASD in their social environment is needed, the similarities in the characteristics of ASD and ADHD regarding problems with social interactions suggest a relationship between the social skills deficits and inattentiveness. Both diagnoses have some neurobiological component, and children with either diagnosis create stress for their parents and teachers.

ATTENTION DEFICIT HYPERACTIVITY DISORDER IN SUB-SAHARAN AFRICA

The diagnosis of ADHD is becoming more common in different African countries, including Nigeria. Adewuya and

Famuyiwa (2007) shed some light on the prevalence of the condition in Nigeria. Although their study conducted in the western part of the country did not represent the entire nation, their findings are significant. They reported the prevalence of ADHD amongst Nigerian primary school students residing in Ilesa, Osun State, in western Nigeria, at 8.7%. This figure for 6- to 12-year-olds is considerably higher than the 1.5% found for children in Ethiopia. The growing population of children with ADHD throughout the world and current research continue to prove that ADHD has no cultural restriction and the condition that was once linked with the Western world (Adewuya & Famuyiwa) has become an international phenomenon.

IMPACT OF ATTENTION DEFICIT HYPERACTIVITY DISORDER ON CHILDREN WITH ASD

Children with ASD also diagnosed with ADHD experience chronic problems with social interaction. The intensity of their social interaction problems is compounded by the fact that ADHD impacts not only the ability to remain attentive to oneself, but also the ability to maintain appropriate social relationships. The child or adolescent with ADHD is usually restless and unable to remain attentive in many ways. Of the different characteristics of ADHD—inattention, hyperactivity, distractibility, and impulsivity—inattention is the predominant characteristic among children also diagnosed with ASD (Gjevik et al., 2011).

Sometimes and in some individuals diagnosed with ASD, the signs and symptoms of inattention and hyperactivity are overt, and at other times and for others the symptoms are less noticeable.

CASE STUDY 3-1

Dami was diagnosed with a mild form of ASD at age 4. Dami is easily frustrated when his needs are not met instantly. He exhibits difficulties staying on topic and most times runs away in the middle of a conversation. He mimics his favorite radio advertisement in an attempt to interrupt the conversations of others or disrupt the activities of others. However, when Dami is redirected, he stays on topic for a few minutes and then . . . he becomes easily distracted again. Dami began receiving speech therapy at age 4 and thus his verbal fluency is about average. Dami is currently 7 years old and his parents are seeking advice on how to help him focus.

In Case Study 3-1 there are three major areas of concern:

1. **Attentiveness:** Dami is experiencing difficulty staying on topic. His attention span seems to be short. Even with redirection, he is able to stay on topic for only a short time.

2. **Distractibility:** Dami not only runs away before a conversation ends, but he usually becomes preoccupied with his own interests such as mimicking a radio advertisement.

3. **Hyperactivity:** Although Dami's symptoms of hyperactivity do not appear intense because he can be easily redirected, he does seem to experience problems staying long in one place.

Based on the short analysis of the case study, inattentiveness, distractibility, and hyperactivity appear to be the major areas of concern for Dami. As you may notice, Dami's symptoms of inattentiveness, hyperactivity, and distractibility are not much different from the symptoms that might be exhibited by a child with ADHD. When Dami is compared to his peers of the same age with a similar diagnosis on the autism spectrum, his behaviors may not appear unusual. It seems fair, therefore, to conclude that Dami's behaviors as indicated above are not enough in themselves to warrant an additional diagnosis of attention deficit hyperactivity disorder. However, it is very important to take the concerns of Dami's parents into consideration. First, the parents are aware that Dami has a diagnosis of ASD. Second, the parents might also be knowledgeable about the symptoms of ADHD. Third, the parents might view Dami's inattention, hyperactivity, and distractibility as increasingly difficult to manage. Fourth, the parents have lived with Dami since he was born and see his current behaviors as out of the norm for him. Given the parents' concerns, a psychologist might need to take a closer look at Dami's behaviors. ADHD symptoms increase the intensity of the social interaction difficulties the child with ASD experiences. That might be the case here.

HASTY CONCLUSIONS AND CONSEQUENCES

In the African culture and particularly within the Nigerian culture, it is very common to hear parents make negative judgments when they are concerned for their children with ASD. Educators also make negative judgments even though they should know better and should be more cognizant of the variations in the presentation of ASD symptoms. On the other hand, when no negative judgments are made, educators tend to minimize the concerns of the parents; this is also common. Look again at the statements of Dami's parents in Case study 3-1:

1. Dami is easily frustrated when his needs are not met.
2. He mimics his favorite radio advertisement in an attempt to interrupt the conversations of others or disrupt the activities of others

The first reaction of some educators to such statements from parents about their child with ASD is to assume that Dami might be manipulating, that he is fully aware of his misconduct. These educators suggest that Dami's parents need to be stricter or firmer with him and possibly punish him when he exhibits such behaviors. Although many in authority might come to the hasty conclusion that Dami is deliberately exhibiting these disruptive behaviors, it is very important that anyone assessing Dami, including parents and educators, not make quick judgments or develop simple hypotheses for Dami's disruptive behaviors without taking into serious consideration the facts that are known about children with ASD. It is a known fact that children with ASD exhibit problems with social interactions and social reciprocity. Hasty conclusions can have serious negative consequences for children with ASD. They can lower their self-esteem, increase the severity of other mental health problems, and exacerbate learning difficulties.

Educators and other professionals in the field of mental health need to take the time to obtain a thorough history of any child with ASD with whom they work, especially if the child's parents express genuine concern. In Nigerian society, parents are often guarded when they report their children's symptoms. The parents might feel shame and guilt if they inform the educator of all the problems their child has. Hasty conclusions or minimizing parent's concerns only increases problems for the child with ASD. Thus, educators must build trust between themselves and the child's parents. On the other hand, if the educator, after obtaining a thorough history from the parents, suspects that poor boundaries between child and parents is a major area that needs to be addressed, the educator should not hold back that or any other concern.

One area of concern in Case Study 3-1 that might be overlooked if hasty conclusions are drawn is Dami's short attention span. A short attention span might indicate a hearing problem. It might also suggest problems with memory and retention, which are characteristic of some children with ASD. In fact, Barnes and colleagues (2008) demonstrated that children diagnosed with ASD typically experience problems with verbal short-term memory. The memory difficulties of children with ASD lie mostly in their inability to remember words or items in the order in which they were communicated to them. This research finding is another reason educators and parents must not jump to the conclusion that the child with ASD is either manipulating or refusing to follow directions. Strategies are available for educators and parents to use to help the child whose short-term memory is significantly impaired.

STRATEGIES FOR IMPROVING AWARENESS IN CHILDREN WITH ASD

The best strategy for improving the attention and focusing skills of children with ASD depend on several variables. Examples of several strategies are presented below.

Build short-term memory. Memory picture game activities can improve short-term memory. Memory picture games consist of pairs of cards, and each card has a picture on one side. The pictures are of familiar objects such as a cat, a dog, a table, or a person wearing a hat. The set of cards contains two of each picture. The players see the pictures, the pictures are turned face down, and then the pictures are scattered around the table. The players watch carefully and try to locate picture pairs. The winner of the game is the person who has found the most paired pictures. For children with ASD, the game doesn't have to last more than 5-10 minutes and the pictures and cards can be hand created by educators or parents.

Simple puzzles are also beneficial in improving short-term memory. However, putting a puzzle together requires lots of patience from both the teacher and the child. As simple as these activities are, when they are repeated consistently for a long period of time, they enable children with ASD to improve their short-term memory. Their social interaction skills will also improve as they continue to participate in these simple activities.

Reduce defiance and distractibility. Understanding the major sources of distraction for the child with ASD is preliminary to minimizing distractibility. Sometimes parents and educators have to validate the object that is the distraction in order to minimize the behavior. For example, if a child with ASD who is easily distracted in conversations because of a compulsion to look at a picture on the wall, the educator might need to validate the picture by mentioning it. Validation might become burdensome for educators and parents because the object is an obsession for the child. When this type of distractibility is frequent, the parent or teacher might need to find an appropriate replacement for the obsession. Ignoring the behavior or the obsessions of the child does not solve the problem. Rather, it intensifies defiance, distractions, and obsessions.

Increase attentiveness. Redirecting children to keep them focused on the subject matter is the most effective method of curbing attentiveness problems. Redirecting can take many forms: verbal instruction, changing the subject of discussion, changing location of activities, discussing rewards and consequences of misbehavior and inattentiveness, or implementing consequences such as time outs or denial of privileges.

CASE STUDY 3-2

Terna is a 9-year-old male with a diagnosis of a moderate form of ASD since age 6. Terna cries a lot and cannot sit still. Terna repeatedly waves his hands within an interval of a few seconds when someone is with him. He has the habit of turning around and gazing at only one portion of the wall when he is being spoken to. Terna is easily distracted by any noise. The only way to keep Terna focused is to ensure that nobody opens the door, no body speaks outside, and no voice is heard inside the room or outside. Terna will not focus in a room with a lot of music gadgets or furniture. In the middle of a somewhat limited and difficult to sustain conversation, he will begin to focus his questions or gaze on the furniture or the music gadgets. He will try to touch them. If it is not the furniture, it is your shoes or your clothing and he will usually want to touch and feel what he is gazing at. His favorite word is "fine." Terna has limited speech and experiences serious difficulties with communication. His parents worry whether Terna will ever be able to speak. His parents, who consider themselves older parents, are concerned for Terna's future when they are deceased. His parents are seeking help for Terna to improve his communication skills, including his inattention and inability to focus. His parents believe that with improved communication and social interaction skills, Terna will be able to manage any uncertainties, and in times of emergencies, others will understand what he is saying and will help him out.

Responsible parents are not only concerned about their children's health and wellbeing; they want to find the best ways to help their children succeed. They think of the future of their children and how their children will be able to live comfortably and independently when they are absent and when age reduces their strength. Terna's parents are responsible parents. The interventions for Terna will vary slightly from those used with Dami. Although both children have diagnosis of ASD, their behaviors differ considerably. Terna seems to experience more problems with attention, focusing, and managing distractions than Dami. Terna's parents are frightened because his inattention, poor communication, distractibility, and difficulties with fine motor skills limit his ability to solve problems and cope with his environment. Further psychological assessment and a more thorough family history are definitely warranted to determine whether a diagnosis of ADHD is in order. From the history given, I would add a provisional diagnosis of ADHD as a secondary diagnosis if Terna were my client.

The purpose here, however, is not to make a diagnosis, but to help you recognize symptoms, understand what they mean, and learn some ways of helping children such as Terna. The cases of Dami and Terna are presented to illustrate the different levels of inattentiveness in children with ASD as exhibited in different behaviors. More thorough histories, examinations, and observations of professionals (psychologists and psychiatrists) are necessary if parents and educators are to provide the best help for their children or adolescents with ASD who exhibit serious deficits in social interaction and social reciprocity.

AGE AND SYMPTOM SEVERITY

To determine the best interventions for children with ASD, parents and educators must look at the relationship between the children's age and the severity of the behaviors they exhibit. The discrepancy between the age of the child and the age at which the behavior is typical indicates the severity of the disorder. In the history presented in Case Study 3-2, Terna is 9 years old and he is described as exhibiting symptoms typical for a 2-year-old male. The 7-year discrepancy is a sign of a severe problem. Terna's parents and educators need to focus on intense interventions. They should obtain a psychiatric and psychological diagnostic assessment. They might also have a primary physician examine Terna to rule out any medical problems that might cause Terna to become more irritable as he grows older. The severity of Terna's communication problem warrants evaluation and probable intervention by a speech therapist.

STRATEGIES FOR IMPROVING SOCIAL INTERACTION SKILLS

Staying with Terna as an example, his parents and educators should obtain a list of his favorite toys or fascinations. He does not seem to hide his fascination or excitement when he approves of an object. The same goes for what irritates him, such as any form of noise. Terna's parents and educators can use the objects that Terna finds fascinating to help him develop a vocabulary of more than one word. It is not unusual for children with ASD to become fixated on a single word or set of words because of their obsessive tendencies. Terna can be taught to say more than "fine" when he describes himself or what he admires.

Children with ASD can be taught to express themselves by using symbols. Write a word and show them symbols to represent the circumstances under which that word is used: the word "hungry" and a picture of food, the word "hurts" and a picture of a sad face. The symbols can be visual or auditory, but in the case of Terna they would probably need to be drawings because noise irritates him. This exercise will help them learn to communicate faster. There is a warning here: although children might be very cooperative when you are teaching them some of the words that are necessary for survival and essential to life such as hungry, wee, bed, hurts, sick, tired, and so on, they might not respond right away by using the words. But if you persist and teach with love, when they are in a situation that requires one of the words, they may surprise you by using the words that you taught them.

Research on improving word learning for children with ASD has shown that the social cues exhibited by the children, such as gazing, facial expressions, and gestures, can be used to produce effective learning experiences (Luyster & Lord, 2009). Luyster and Lord described the "follow up labeling" method of teaching words to children with ASD. In this method, the child holds up a toy or other object and both the teacher and the student label the object verbally. For as long as the child is focused on holding the object, the name of the object is repeated. The expectation is that as a result of saying and hearing the label associated with the object while paying attention to it, the child will learn the label and is able to name the object later. The "follow up labeling" method of teaching might not be new to educators, but the point of reiterating it here is to show that the assumed weakness of the child with ASD, such as gazing, repetitive (obsessive) behavior, or unusual facial expression, becomes of great benefit and a very helpful tool that can be used to improve the child's learning abilities.

IMPROVING UNDERSTANDING OF BEHAVIOR PATTERNS IN CHILDREN WITH ASD WITH ADHD SYMPTOMS

Individuals diagnosed with ASD are unique, and individualized measures are necessary for effective management of their symptoms. The case studies of Dami and Terna are good examples of the uniqueness of children with ASD. Both children have a diagnosis of ASD and both exhibit some problems with attentiveness, distractibility, and focusing. However, the severity of the symptoms varies in the two children. When exploring ways to help children like these, the predominant question is: "What should we look for when it comes to attentiveness, distractibility, hyperactivity, and ASD?" These are my suggestions:

1. Before parents begin to panic, they should evaluate the degree of inattentiveness their children are exhibiting and compare it to the attentiveness of other children of the same age and condition. The severity of the

symptoms of inattention and distractibility will determine the type of strategies that should be implemented.
2. Parents or caregivers should also evaluate the impact
    of the inattentiveness and the distractibility on the chil-
    dren's ability to accomplish independent living tasks
    such as taking showers or bathing, eating, playing,
    cleaning, and washing dishes. When inattentiveness
    and distractibility seriously hinder the development of
    the children's independent living skills, more behavioral
    and psychological intervention is required. Educators
    can help the parents in this matter because the school
    has some responsibility for fostering positive behaviors.
    Please note that children with ASD with serious medical
    or neurological conditions such as cerebral palsy, Rett's
    syndrome, Fragile X syndrome, frequent seizures, or
    severe motor or gait problems might have to depend
    on others for the rest of their lives. However, many chil-
    dren with ASD and no co-morbid medical conditions are
    teachable and they are capable of independent living.

The relationship between the inattentiveness and distractibility experienced by children with ASD and problem behaviors
such as defiance and oppositional defiance disorder has been
documented by several researchers (Adewuya & Famuyiwa,
2007; Gjevik et al., 2011). When the inattentiveness and distractibility of the child with ASD becomes associated with problematic behaviors, the method of reducing the problematic behaviors is more behavior focused. There are different methods

of addressing problematic behaviors in children with ASD. The behavior modification plan discussed in part 2 of this book entails obtaining a comprehensive evaluation of the child's pattern of inattentiveness and distractions, and this requires taking into consideration what I call "antecedents" and "succedents." Behaviors provide the child with ASD some gratification, either positive or negative. For example, inattentive and easily distracted teenagers with ASD sometimes find it unpleasant to go to school because they receive reprimands from the teacher. When it is time to go to school, they may throw a serious tantrum characterized by cries, wailing, and refusing to eat to the extent that their frustrated parent(s) may let them stay home. In such an instance, there are factors that preceded the behavior, causing the child to avoid school (antecedents) as well as benefits that occur after the behavior, such as staying home instead of going to school (succedents). Understanding the antecedents and succedents of problem behaviors will go a long way toward developing an appropriate behavior modification plan. Whatever behavior modification strategy is developed for the child with ASD and coexisting diagnosis of ADHD, the intervention must be repeated multiple times for effectiveness. For children and adolescents with ASD who are inattentive or easily distracted, strategies must be repeated often and for long periods of time to produce lasting change.

NEUROSCIENCE RESEARCH ON BRAIN FUNCTION

The similarity in brain functioning in children diagnosed with ASD and children diagnosed with ADHD are of interest to many educators and parents. It is thus relevant for parents and educators in Nigeria to know that this very interesting scientific research is still ongoing. Researchers such as Lionel et al. (2011) have studied the brains of individuals with ASD and individuals with ADHD, examining the lobes that control impulsivity/inattentiveness, odd behaviors, and communication difficulties. In an attempt to prove that both disorders might be caused by the same gene or brain malfunction, they have found some relationships between the two disorders.

CASE STUDY 3-3

Nzo is a 15-year-old male with a normal physical appearance and excellent speech, good in verbal and expressive language. Nzo is the youngest of two male children. Both Nzo's parents are secondary school teachers and both described Nzo as a "busy body" since age 2. Nzo is currently in primary five and experiences academic problems. Nzo is not in a special school. He is often teased at school and does not have friends. Although Nzo experiences significant difficulties maintaining friendships, he has no difficulties approaching any person, be it an-other student, a teacher, or a passer-by, to begin a friendly conversation. Nzo has always believed that he will grow up to be in the Nigerian army or navy. Nzo will cry or throw tantrums if his parents do not buy him a toy gun or a toy military car with siren. Nzo will line up his toy vehicles and guns in his room at night, pretending that he is at war, with no lights on in the room, and he will crawl on the floor. Sometimes Nzo will have a flashlight or torchlight on top of the bed while pretending to be at war. In recent months, Nzo has been running away from home and taking to the streets. His parents are experienc-ing frustration and anxiety over Nzo's choices. Nzo has continually indicated that he is tired of living in the same place and needs to move in with military people. Nzo does not seem to understand that he is not old enough to enlist. In recent months, his parents have found Nzo crawling on the floor stating that he is in search of his enemies; he can do this several times during the day. Nzo has re-cently declined to complete his school work. He has been tutored at home due to his parents' feelings of shame over his behaviors. His personal tutor of 9 months has time and again informed his ambitious parents that Nzo is not capable of understanding his math and English. His tu-tor further stated that Nzo is playful and easily distracted.

His tutor said Nzo has problems sitting still for more than 30 minutes. The tutor is currently expressing high levels of frustration and has decided to resign unless the parents take Nzo to see a physician, stating, "This child is not well."

As odd as this case might sound, there are parents in Nigeria who will identify with this story. The major question that such parents are confronted with is how to help their children who refuse to learn despite all the resources they have invested in the children's learning. In this case study, Nzo seems to have coped well for many years, he has no external physical malformation or troubling symptoms, he attends a regular school, and his communication skills are not impaired. Thus, many parents and educators in Nigeria would have difficulty believing that Nzo has psychological problems. A typical description of Nzo in the Nigerian context would be "stubborn and wicked." Well, let us not condemn Nzo. Yes!! Nzo might not present with the classic ASD symptoms. Yet, consider the following behaviors Nzo have displayed that are, in fact, symptoms of ASD:

1. **Problems with social interaction.** He has no friends and experiences problems maintaining friendships. But he has no difficulties initiating conversation and maintaining rapport with a stranger.

2. **Odd behaviors:** He is fascinated with toy guns and sleeps with these guns. He pretends to be fighting wars in his room although he is 15 years old. He cries and throws a

tantrum if he is not given a toy gun. He wants to move in with military people, possibly at their barracks.

3. **Odd and repetitive behavior patterns:** He crawls on the floor in search of his enemies.

4. **Learning difficulties:** He does not focus. He is not doing well academically, even with a private tutor.

5. **Attention problems/distractibility:** He has difficulty focusing and remaining attentive. He is reported as restless and has been a "busy body" from a young age.

6. **Defiance:** Nzo is refusing to attend school. He becomes emotional and disruptive if asked to attend school. He runs away from home and takes to the streets.

7. **Inappropriate boundaries and immaturity:** Nzo appears quite immature and personal boundaries are indeed a problem.

If a more comprehensive psychological assessment were completed on Nzo, it is possible that more bizarre behaviors would be observed and reported by his parents. Cases such as Nzo's are actually quite difficult to explain to parents who are uninformed or have little experience managing children or adolescents with developmental disorders.

POSSIBLE HYPOTHESES

Developmental psychologists often construct different hypotheses to help them get a clear picture of a person's problematic behaviors. Some of the hypotheses developed for Nzo might be as follows:

1. Nzo is experiencing problems learning probably because he has not fully comprehended the basics of math and the English Language. Thus, learning has become frustrating and burdensome for him.

2. The frustration and difficulties that Nzo is experiencing are manifested in his choices of running away from home and in his irrational and increased interest in becoming a military man.

3. Nzo's odd behaviors of fascination with wars and crawling like a child might be attributed to some developmental or other psychiatric problems.

4. Nzo may actually be thinking of his future and concluding that since his academic performance is poor, he may do well to enlist in the military.

5. The defiance that Nzo is exhibiting as seen in his refusal to complete his school work might be a result of low self-concept; perhaps has been confronted with demeaning statements.

I encourage teachers in Nigeria to develop hypotheses when they are confronted with difficult case scenarios. An appropriate hypothesis may be used to discover and address the causes of problematic behaviors in children. A good hypothesis coupled with a very thorough history may lead to the development of the best education and learning plan for the child who exhibits problematic behaviors. Individualized learning plans are necessary when children with ASD exhibit serious symptoms of ADHD. In a case like Nzo's, effective intervention strategies will require the involvement of a psychologist and/or a psychiatrist because of the oddness of the behaviors.

It is an established fact that inattentiveness and distraction can coexist with ASD. What is most important is that parents and educators attempt to understand the severity of the ADHD symptoms in their children with ASD and how those symptoms impact the functioning of their children. For some children, behavioral interventions are enough to reduce the ADHD symptoms to a manageable level, but for others, psychiatric or psychotropic medications might be necessary. Whichever is the case, parents and educators should always evaluate the reason for their choice of interventions, making sure the purpose is to improve the wellbeing of the child rather than enhance their own comfort. In the case of Nzo, without appropriate interventions he might end up becoming a street child, a drug addict or alcoholic, a member of local motor park thugs, or a drifter.

The adage frequently repeated in Nigeria that "nobody seeks the help of a doctor when he has no illness" could easily have been applied to Nzo. But if it had been, his opportunity to have specialized and individualized training in mathematics and language would have been lost. Yes, people seek positive interventions and strategies only when problems exist. However, sometimes, when proper interventions are not implemented in a timely manner parents lose their power to control their child's behavior and chaos and sadness follow in the short term. But parents need to take hold of hope and do what is best for their children. Whenever parents or guardians realize that they have failed to take certain steps or implemented major techniques in the raising of their child, they should not be afraid to begin afresh. Parents in Nigeria, there are a lot of help available. You are not alone. So cast aside the shame and seek help for the sake of your children's successful future.

4

ENCOUNTERING EMOTIONAL DIFFICULTIES

The emotional difficulties children and adolescents with ASD encounter can be detrimental to their physical and psychological health. Therefore, parents, caregivers, and educators need to have basic methods of identifying the signs and symptoms of emotional problems in children with ASD. The term "emotional difficulties or problems" is used in its broadest sense in this book and includes a variety of mood disorders. Mood disorders are sometimes referred to as affective disorders; they include depression, anxiety, bipolar disorder, and others. Emotional difficulties or mood disorders are not the feelings children with ASD experience on a daily basis; they are serious conditions.

Differentiating between anxiety and depression in children with ASD is difficult because the physical manifestations of these conditions tend to overlap. Tantrums, frequent outbursts of anger, difficulties with sleep, problems with appetite, isolation, agitation, low tolerance for frustration, and crying spells are some of the frequently observed signs of both depression and anxiety. The presentation of these symptoms in children is covert (Ebesutani et al., 2012; Muris & Meesters, 2002). In Nigeria, as long as children with ASD do not have fevers or physical problems, their anxiety or depression symptoms are likely to be ignored or mistaken for disobedience. Anxiety and depression can co-occur in children with ASD or anxiety can precede depression. Whatever is the case, parents, caregivers, and educators need to be alert to the signs of depression and anxiety so they can explore what is causing the child to have emotional problems so they can prevent them and, if possible, eradicate them.

THE EXPERIENCE OF EMOTIONAL DIFFICULTIES IN CHILDREN AND ADOLESCENTS WITH ASD

In children or adolescents with ASD residing in Nigeria, depression and anxiety might initially manifest as physical problems. They might complain of frequent headaches, loss of appetite, fear that they have malaria, ongoing fatigue, and difficulties with vision. The depression and anxiety can also be masked, the symptoms such as blank or neutral facial expression, social withdrawal, and engaging in self-injurious behaviors attributed to the characteristics of ASD (Hillier, Fish, Siegel, & Beversdorf, 2011).

As children with ASD develop into adolescents, they tend to become conscious of how they are viewed by their peers and of their roles in society, and this awareness can give rise to or intensify emotional difficulties. Moreover, the experience of depression and anxiety during adolescence is more problematic for boys than for girls in Nigeria (Egbikuadje, 2005). It is not unusual for children with ASD, especially males, to become emotionally distraught because of their developmental disability as they become adolescents and begin to think of their future. Many adolescent females with ASD cope by becoming more interested in activities and materials that enhance their physical appearance than in how they can or cannot contribute to their family; they appear to become egocentric. With males, however, as they enter adolescence, they begin to realize that instead of eventually becoming caretakers of their parents and younger siblings, they are going to be cared for by their parents and siblings, probably their whole lifetime. Not surprisingly, more adolescent males than adolescent females suffer from depression or anxiety in the Nigerian society.

Interestingly, adolescents with ASD with higher intellectual abilities experience more emotional problems (Attwood, 2008; Hillier et al., 2011). The reason is that they continue to have difficulties fitting in with their peers and they are aware of differences between them and others. Although adolescents with ASD with higher intellectual functioning might attempt to hide their symptoms of oddness and obsessions when they are with their peers, they continue to face rejection and neglect. Consequently, they might not want to be around their peers for fear of being ridiculed, and self-pity becomes a way of life. Adolescents with ASD who are not intellectually challenged struggle with their tendency to define themselves in terms of how they are viewed by their peers. Many times, their very low self-concepts keep them from believing in themselves and accepting themselves for who they are and what they can achieve. Therefore, the anxiety experienced by the child with ASD is characterized mainly by excessive worries and fears and anxiety can be the result of specific trauma; the depression they experience is characterized by agitation, increasing feelings of sadness, lack of motivation, feelings of fatigue, and feelings of hopelessness. The rate at which the depression and the anxiety experience of the child or adolescent with ASD progresses from a mild to a serious problem can vary or change quickly if positive remedies are not put in place on time.

CULTURAL FACTORS AND EMOTIONAL EXPRESSIONS

In the Nigerian culture, males are expected to be brave and not express emotions in public. In a study of adolescent males' and females' experiences of death depression in the Niger Delta region of Nigeria, Egbikuadje (2005) found out that although more adolescent females expressed their emotions and fears, more adolescent males refrained from showing their emotions and expressed minimal fears. Adolescent males with

ASD experience higher depression and anxiety than females because of their tendency to keep their emotions in check until they take a toll on their bodies. Parents, caregivers, and educators are encouraged, therefore, not to ignore any change in the lives of children with ASD.

The ability of the adolescent male with ASD to deal with fears and frustrations is hindered by his fear of not being viewed as strong and courageous. Although it is important for adolescent males with ASD to grow up feeling courageous and emotionally strong, parents and educators need to inform them that in times of extreme emotional difficulties they should either freely discuss their problems with their parents or close family members or seek professional help. Furthermore, when communication through the use of words is very difficult for the child or adolescent with ASD, it is up to the parent and the educator to be cognizant of the different gestures the child or adolescent uses to express different emotions. In the Nigerian culture, it is very easy for parents and educators to neglect the emotions of children with ASD. They reason that as long as children are physically healthy and most of their basic needs and necessities are met, they should not have any reason to be worried or depressed.

Although the discussion of depression and anxiety in this book focuses on conditions resulting from environmental factors, it is important to note that depression and anxiety can be pathological or genetic. If children or adolescents with ASD in Nigeria have their needs provided for and show signs of worry and sadness, they are usually viewed as unappreciative. Inasmuch as parents and educators desire validation from their children or students with ASD for their good work, they should not view negative emotional expressions from the children or students only in terms of how dissatisfied the children are.

RELIGIOSITY AND EMOTIONAL EXPRESSIONS

Overall, Nigerians handle the symptoms of depression and anxiety better than many others because of their religious inclinations. Their concepts of faith and hope are remarkable. However, there are numerous Nigerians who view depression and anxiety as stress driven; their desire to reduce the stress through medications is sometimes extreme. Children or adolescents who were brought up with strong faith and religious values are expected to accept the values of their parents and act accordingly. In severe cases, it seems unreasonable to assume that children and adolescents with ASD will necessarily understand and accept faith and religious values with the same fervor as their parents. Consequently, considering the different levels of severity of ASD symptoms, more scientific studies are needed to evaluate the impact of religiosity on the ability of children and adolescents with ASD to express their negative emotions. Do they really understand the concept of religiosity?

PHYSICAL AGGRESSION, VERBAL OUTBURSTS, AND NIGHTMARES

Parents and educators monitor their children and adolescents with ASD to ensure that the symptoms that suggest emotional difficulties are under control. Symptoms of depression and anxiety are difficult to observe in children with communication difficulties and in students with lower intellectual abilities. In addition, children and adolescents who have learned to communicate how they feel to their parents and their educators have probably also learned better ways to resolve their internal conflicts of feeling different from their peers. Consequently, although they might show signs of emotional difficulties at different times in their lives, they have a better handle on their negative thoughts and they might be open to seeking help for their emotional problems. Parents who have sought help for their children from a very young age, have maintained positive interaction with them, and have been integral parts of their lives from the time they suspected that their children were developmentally delayed tend to have better rapport with their children. These children that maintain close relationships with their parents tend to cope better during periods of emotional difficulties.

Physical expression of emotional difficulties—aggression, agitation, and verbal outbursts—are not uncommon in children in Nigeria. Usually, however, the child with ASD experiencing serious emotional problems is also experiencing rejection and neglect. It is therefore important to monitor the daily activities of children and adolescents with ASD more closely when their symptoms of emotionality are overwhelming and obvious. Increase in aggression, increased agitation, and frequent nightmares in children or adolescents with ASD should always be taken seriously. Children and adolescents with ASD frequently express their frustrations and intense disapproval through aggression and agitation during the day and nightmares at night.

Let me illustrate aggression in a child with ASD with a story. Although hypothetical, the story is close to reality. It will help you understand emotional difficulties and their expression in aggression, verbal outbursts, and nightmares. Perhaps more importantly, it will show why parents, caregivers, siblings, and educators need to monitor children with ASD more closely when they are becoming increasingly needy.

This is the story of a 7-year-old boy with ASD described as mean, aggressive, annoying, and having difficulty managing his anger. He has severe motor difficulties as well as very limited speech. This young boy was taken to see a psychotherapist because of his aggression, which caused his brother to have stitches in his forehead. This young child was under the care of a paid home health nanny 6 days a week because both parents work 5 days a week and his only brother (12 years old) attends school 5 days a week. The child, who became so aggressive that he threw a chair at his brother, was diagnosed with severe depression.

After a couple of sessions of psychotherapy and behavior consultation, the therapists discovered that this young child with ASD had been starved daily by the nanny for more than 3 months. Unknown to his parents, the nanny was throwing away his meals every day. The young child had attempted with his limited speech to report his feelings of hunger, pain, anger, and sadness, but no one understood him. When he watched his brother eat, he cried and stretched his hands forward as a gesture to be fed. His brother either ignored him, stating, "You ate yours already" or obliged him by sharing his meals. Also during psychotherapy the young child appeared significantly dehydrated.

His parents' response to the psychotherapist's concern was that their child's sleep was limited due to his intense feelings of fear at night and also fears that in the morning he would be left alone in the house. His parents stated that sometimes their child yells in his sleep. His parents justified their working and leaving him by saying, "We can't help him if we don't work." Although the parents were caring for their child in the way they deemed best, it appeared that they trusted the nanny. Thus, the nanny had not been supervised or questioned. The psychotherapist described the young child as significantly depressed and determined that the depression was the result of ongoing feelings of rejection through starvation. The child's growing depression resulting from maltreatment extended beyond feelings of anger towards his nanny; he was also angry towards all the members of his family.

The parents of the 7-year-old child were fatigued at the end of the day's work and also at the end of the week, and their fatigue kept them from recognizing their son's frustrations as abnormal for him. His brother, who was older than the boy, could not figure out the reason for the sudden change in his temperament and behaviors. How frustrating it must have been for this 7-year-old! This story illustrates the value in seeking professional help outside of the family; positive results often follow involvement of professionals. The good news about depression and other emotional problems is that the experiences can be minimized if managed correctly. New findings regarding the causes of the depression in the child with ASD are offering promise that depression symptoms can be reduced.

THE EXPERIENCE OF GENERALIZED ANXIETY DISORDER

Anxiety disorders and other psychiatric disorders are more prevalent among children with ASD than in the normal population (Matson & Sturmey, 2011). The occurrence of anxiety symptoms has been documented for children with ASD with high intellectual abilities as well as those with low intellectual abilities (Strang et al., 2012). Children with the diagnosis of both ADHD and ASD experience more anxiety than children with ASD alone.

Anxiety is manifested in a variety of symptoms. Anxiety is typically characterized by the presence of increased fears regarding certain places or objects. Generalized anxiety disorder is very common among children with ASD who attend school (Guttmann-Steinmetz, Gadow, DeVincent, & Crowell, 2010). Children with ASD experience more anxiety in the school environment than any other place (Gadow, De Vincent, & Pomeroy, 2006). One reason for the high level of anxiety at school is probably that the school environment requires social interaction and communication. Another reason is the association of school with generalized anxieties that are characterized by phobias, or fears of specific objects or experiences (Gjevik et al., 2011; Guttmann-Steinmetz et al.). Although there may be a relationship between obsessive behaviors and repetitive but odd patterns of behaviors and the ongoing difficulties with social interactions for the child with ASD, there is no conclusive evidence that children or adolescents with ASD are anxious because they are attempting to avoid social interactions (Gjevik et al.). However, the need for social interaction is one of the pressures of the school environment, and pressure creates fear in individuals with ASD.

ANXIETY AND SOCIAL INTERACTION DEFICITS

How do environmental pressures create fear in the child with ASD? One environmental pressure may come from the children's parents. Well-meaning parents attempt to boost the self-esteem of their children who do not have the intellectual ability to do certain academic tasks by telling them they are capable of competing with their counterparts in the classroom. However, they overlook the consequences of the pressure their well-intentioned actions place on the child with ASD. When children with ASD do not feel they are as competent as their parents led them to believe, they begin to experience fear. Although the parent's strategies to boost their children's self-esteem and academic achievement are not totally out of place, parents need to be careful of the extent they go in trying to help their children achieve academically. There has to be a balance between validation and disapproval of the child's academic achievements. Parents and guardians should refrain from making comparisons between their children and their friends' children, as is commonly done in the Nigerian culture. Such comparisons can be detrimental to the psychological health of the child or adolescent with ASD, who is already psychologically fragile. On the contrary, for children with ASD with intellectual disabilities, parents, guardians, and educators should take positive action to help them discover their talents. Each child has a unique skill and sometimes that skill is not readily observed. But with ongoing positive support from parents and educators, children with ASD can discover their unique skills.

Another environmental pressure comes from the behaviors that are characteristic of ASD, including difficulties with communication and social interaction, failure to establish appropriate social boundaries, exhibition of odd behaviors, obsessive patterns of behaviors, and some stereotypical behaviors such as smiling inconsistently or frequent hand waving or waggling. As children with ASD with no intellectual disabilities or other mental health conditions grow into adolescence, their knowledge that they have these mannerisms may cause them shame. By adolescence they are cognizant of who they are and how they are in comparison with their peers and they feel that they are different. It is therefore the responsibility of the educator, the school guidance counselor, and especially the parent and the guardian to help them feel great with themselves. The experience of shame and a low self-concept should never be allowed to permit a child's anxiety symptoms to develop into a pathological disorder. If their fears and worries are addressed in the early stages and they are given the necessary help, children with ASD can be prevented from developing symptoms that call for a diagnosable condition of anxiety disorder.

Some of the other environmental factors that can contribute to the development of anxiety symptoms in children with ASD are the experience of being teased and mocked by peers in the neighborhood; being ignored by parents, educators, siblings, caregivers, or guardians; and being frequently isolated or left alone in the home because the parents or their siblings do not want to be faced with the added responsibility of caring for them in social gatherings. Although some children with ASD might not appear intellectually capable, they have very sensitive emotions. Rejection and neglect add significantly to the emotional difficulties they experience. They might pretend to be scared when what they really need is attention. It is up to parents and educators to recognize and identify the underlying reason for the attention seeking behavior of the child with ASD.

DIAGNOSABLE CONDITIONS OF ANXIETY AND DEPRESSION

Considering the cultural variability in the presentation of both anxiety and depression symptoms in children with ASD, parents and professionals cannot rely only on the guidelines provided in the International Classification of Diseases codes or the *Diagnostic and Statistical Manual of Mental Disorders*. Although these diagnostic guidelines are helpful as starting points, mental health clinicians cannot ignore the degree of impact of the emotional problem of the child on their home, school, and social environment.

CASE STUDY 4-1

Omo was diagnosed with ASD at age 11 and he did not begin any formal education until that age. Omo has never lived in a home with educated parents or adults. Omo is the first of three children and the only male child in the home. Both his parents are traders at the local market. Omo understands his local language only and does not have any knowledge of English, which is the language used in school. When he first arrived at school, he appeared scared and was much older than his peers in the same classroom. Omo does not speak at school and rarely engages in play with peers during recess. Omo's frequent crying spells create confusion in the teacher, who does not know if Omo is hungry or is having problems adjusting to the school environment. Omo does not smile and has irregular eye contact. When his parents were informed of his behaviors at school, they responded: "He is always like that... since he was born. Nothing else to do... just to pray... thank you!" When Omo was on a week's break from school, his crying spells and isolation behaviors intensified. When Omo returned to school after the week-long mid-term break, he began defecating and urinating on himself in the class-room. He seemed afraid all the time. He increasingly ex-hibited repetitive behavior, moving his neck rhythmically to the right. Omo's ability to focus in the classroom has deteriorated, and he cries when peers try to help him. Re-cently, and probably after about 2 months at school, his parents went to the school to tell the class teacher just this: "Our son is getting worse. What is happening with this school? He was not like this before he started school." His parents threatened to withdraw their son from the special school because he was not getting better and they were having more difficulty focusing on their trade.

Although the history given in Case Study 4-1 is scant, these remarks or observations from Omo's parents are troubling:

1. Omo's parents, who did not initially view their son's symptoms as out of the norm, became concerned about their son's symptoms after a few months of school.

2. Omo's parents were not specific in their explanation of what they considered "normal" behavior when they were approached by the school teacher.

3. Omo's parents viewed the school environment as creat-ing problems for their son and they seem to attribute their son's increasing symptoms to his experience at school.

EMOTIONAL DIFFICULTIES, SOCIAL INTERACTION, AND THE SCHOOL ENVIRONMENT

In Case Study 4-1, the following emotional difficulties experienced by Omo are evident:

1. Omo appeared scared when he first arrived at school.
2. He has ongoing crying spells that create confusion in the mind of the teacher.
3. He feels fear when he is at school.
4. He resents help from his peers at school.
5. He refuses to smile and he does not engage in play at school.

In addition to the emotional difficulties Omo exhibited at home and at school, once he started school he began experiencing increased symptoms in these areas:

1. More repetitive and obsessive behaviors such as rhythmically moving his neck towards his right
2. Social isolation
3. Encopresis (defecating on himself) and enuresis (urinating on himself)
4. Inability to stay focused; attention difficulties

Strategically, the teacher should evaluate Omo's readiness for school. A major problem Omo faces in school is the language. Omo does not understand the English language and his parents do not appear educated enough to be able to teach him English at home. It is reasonable to assume that the language barrier is a significant factor in Omo's adjustment difficulties. Second, it is not unusual for children with ASD with significant emotional problems resulting from adjustment difficulties to experience increased anxiety when they are on a week's break from school. Third, Omo resents having to go to school and he exhibits his dissatisfaction with the school environment by his emotional symptoms. His fears during the break from school that he might be sent back to the school might be impacting his social interaction skills and his obsessive patterns of behaviors. Fourth, it is not surprising that Omo feels intimidated at school. He is much older than his classmates and he is new to the school. His behaviors might be the result of very poor self-esteem, which in fact correlates significantly with the experience of anxiety and depression in children with ASD. Educators who are confronted with the types of problems seen in this case study or who suspect that a student in their classroom might be having serious difficulties adjusting to the school environment are encouraged to explore the following options:

1. Obtain a thorough family history that includes a schedule of activities in the home to find out if the child is experiencing isolation or neglect in the home. Omo's teacher should find out if Omo has any siblings and should note that his parents are traders. They should ask with whom Omo stays after school and if he goes to the store with his parents. What does Omo do and where does he go to after school?

2. Explore with the child's parents what has changed in the child's life since the child began school, including but

not limited to the child's daily schedule. Any change can significantly impact the life of a student with ASD.

3. Obtain a thorough history of some of Omo's behaviors prior to the time he began school, including the times he met his developmental milestones. Ask questions about his ability to use the toilet and if he has any problems with urinary incontinence. It is interesting that Omo is defecating in the classroom. Urinary incontinence is not uncommon for children with severe developmental disability. However, if Omo has been potty trained (which we don't know), his behaviors of defecating and urinating in the classroom at age 11 indicates a huge problem. These behaviors make Omo's condition more complicated.

4. Educate the parents on some of the problems that children with ASD commonly experience in the school environment. When parents are uneducated, sending their children with ASD to school can be quite challenging. However, teachers should have a simple discussion at the parents' level of understanding. Educators want to avoid situations in which uneducated parents misperceive their messages as meaning that their children have the worst behaviors in the classroom.

RESOLVING EMOTIONAL DIFFICULTIES IN CHILDREN AND ADOLESCENTS WITH ASD

In most cases of children with ASD with emotional difficulties, the history a teacher receives is usually incomplete.

Teachers need to inform the children's parents or caregivers that providing a complete and thorough history facilitates a more definite diagnosis, which allows for good strategic treatment plans. As emphasized previously, many children with ASD experiencing emotional difficulties have low self-esteem. Children and adolescents with ASD in Nigeria endure a lot of criticism and frequent mocking and teasing from their peers. Many of the frustrations they experience from being developmentally delayed can be alleviated by the love and the acceptance they receive from their family members. The love and acceptance from their family members might be the only assurance of their worth they have in their entire lives. Because the emotional difficulties children with ASD experience is a function of their environment, it is very important for parents to continually assure their children that they are safe even if the parents are absent for a number of hours or a few days. The trust children with ASD are able to place in their environment is the result of the combination of these factors: the degree of assurance they receive from their parents, the feelings of acceptance they perceive from their teachers, and the degree of acceptance they perceive from their peers at school.

5

ATYPICAL AFFINITIES

Time and again, Nigerians have referred to individuals who have ASD as "mad," "crazy," "witches," or "curses." Little did they know that these children suffered from what was later found to be autism spectrum disorder. The tendency for family members to want to hide their "strange" child from the view of friends, neighbors, family members and others in the community was very strong due to the significant stigma associated with ASD. Parents who thought negatively of their children and tried to hide them, do not feel guilty just yet. Be consoled by the fact that early researchers first described ASD as "infantile psychosis" (Kolvin, 1972). Even educated scientist in the early days mistook ASD for psychosis. Nonetheless, to think today of children with ASD as schizophrenics or psychotics is flawed. Current medical research examining the similarities and dissimilarities between ASD and schizophrenia has identified key differences in terms of the functions and the anatomy of the brains of people with ASD and schizophrenics (e.g., Sugranyes, Kyriakopoulos, Corrigall, Taylor, & Frangou, 2011). Researchers continue to investigate the executive functioning of the brain of both people with ASD and schizophrenics, probably because more information in this area might create more opportunities for experimenting on psychopharmacological treatment opportunities or cure options for ASD.

ASD, PSYCHOSIS, AND STIGMA

The discrimination children with ASD have experienced over the years can be partly attributed to the belief among some that children with ASD are psychotic. Consequently, everyone does not understand that many people with ASD are capable of becoming educated, learning vocational trades, and living comfortable lives. Some of the stereotypical behaviors that cause many Nigerians to view individuals with ASD as psychotics are rhythmically banging hands or objects on a table, turning on and switching off the lights in the house, running back and forth in the house, twitching their neck in one direction, being preoccupied with one part of an object and gazing fixedly at it, fascination with certain body parts that might be deemed inappropriate, rocking their bodies back and forth to the extent that observers are disturbed, walking on tiptoes, arranging objects or pictures in a specific order and rhythmically, and standing near a stranger too close for comfort.

Some of the restricted and repetitive patterns of behaviors exhibited by children with ASD have also been observed in individuals diagnosed with schizophrenia, tic disorders, cerebral palsy, Down syndrome, Fragile X syndrome, and Parkinson's disease (Leekam, Prior, & Uljarevic, 2011). These behaviors include rhythmic body movements and rhythmic sound production. In comparing the behaviors of children with ASD and children with other mental disorders, Leekam et al. found that repetitive and stereotypical behavior patterns were more frequent in children with ASD than in children with any other classification of mental disorders such as schizophrenia. Although calling for more research to definitively determine the causes of the odd behavior patterns, Leekam et al. attributed the repetitive and stereotypical behavior patterns in people diagnosed with ASD to the complex activities involved in the interactions of the neurobiological, social, behavioral, genetic, and cognitive facets of the human person.

Genetic factors appear to be involved in both schizophrenia and ASD, although the research about genetics as a cause of developmental disabilities is controversial and inconclusive (McAlonan et al., 2008; Toal et al., 2009). Some researchers believe strongly that the origin of the disorders is genetic and others assert that ASD is the result of either some vaccine administered to the child before the age of 3 years or environmental toxins (Desoto & Hirlan, 2007). Furthermore, some neuroscientists suggest that the executive functioning part of the brain of the person diagnosed with ASD is the same as for the schizophrenic. When neuroscientists find similarities in symptoms of different disorders, they tend to capitalize on the similarities to find cures. Thus researchers such as Possey and McDougle (2000) experimented with antipsychotics on people diagnosed with ASD.

Despite the use of antipsychotics on individuals with ASD, ASD should not be mistaken for schizophrenia. Professionals must conduct appropriate psychological and psychiatric assessments in order to confirm a diagnosis of schizophrenia in an individual with ASD. Parents learning of the possibility of a connection between ASD and psychosis by reading this book should not panic; panic is unproductive and detrimental to the psychological and physical health of the child with ASD. As you may well know, some individuals diagnosed with ASD have co-existing conditions of psychosis, and they exhibit symptoms comparable to what is observed in schizophrenics. If a parent or educator suspects this is the case with a particular child, they should refer the child with ASD for a thorough psychiatric evaluation. It is not helpful to observe symptoms and refer to the child as "crazy"; rather, the focus should be on obtaining early treatment interventions for the affected child.

Considering the abundance of stigma in the Nigerian culture against individuals with ASD, parents and educators need to know some basics about the differences in the characteristics of schizophrenia and of ASD. The classic symptoms of schizophrenia observed in the Nigerian culture, and clearly spelled out in the International Classification of Diseases code, include the following: hallucinations, paranoia, disorganized behaviors such as smiling to oneself, and bizarre delusions. The symptoms manifested by the schizophrenic can be distinguished from the symptoms of ASD in four points. First, the hallucinations experienced by the schizophrenic cannot be mistaken for the ASD individuals' obsession tendencies such as fixation on a particular piece of music on a particular radio station or washing one plate or dish for more than 20 minutes. The music on the radio station and the activity of washing the dish or plate are real activities; hallucinations are not real. Second, the bizarre delusions of schizophrenics can range from believing a bug is crawling on their skin, or believing they are God, to believing they have the power to conquer the world with their tongue. On the contrary, individuals with ASD do not have bizarre delusions unless they have a coexisting psychotic disorder such as schizophrenia. Third, although individuals with ASD and individuals with schizophrenia have difficulties with social interactions, their difficulties are different. The individuals with ASD prefer isolative play and have to learn to socialize with their peers; those with schizophrenia do not necessarily enjoy isolative play, but prefer to stay to themselves, probably because of the "voices" or hallucinations that impact their processing or thinking skills. Fourth, although some of the symptoms of ASD such as social interaction skills deficits can be minimized or improved over the course of time, the symptoms can be viewed as a "way of life" for the person with ASD. Schizophrenics, on the other hand, might have lucid moments or moments of sanity, but their thoughts are distorted, and the condition is more of an illness than a way of life. Schizophrenia is not readily diagnosed in toddlers or other children, but the symptoms of ASD appear in early childhood.

The stigmatizing belief in Nigeria that ASD is "childhood madness" or is the result of a curse or witchcraft needs to be changed. Educators, parents, and other professionals in Nigeria should take up the task of educating the public about ASD when the need arises so that children with ASD can get the help they deserve from a young age. Although some children with ASD have improved when treated with medications used in the treatment of schizophrenia or other psychotic disorders, this fact alone is not sufficient to justify equating ASD to "childhood madness."

MEDICATIONS AND ASD

Atypical antipsychotics that are effective in the treatment of psychotic symptoms such as schizophrenia have also been found effective in the treatment of some of the symptoms of ASD (Julien, Advokat, & Comaty, 2011). The purpose of discussing medications and ASD in this chapter is to make clear to parents and educators that medications should not be prescribed because a child has been diagnosed with ASD or because the child with ASD is becoming a burden to parents or caregivers. The proper use of medications, including antipsychotics, is to alleviate in children with ASD the symptoms that are causing them to inflict serious harm on themselves or others. Although Aripiprazole (Abilify) has been used, Risperidone (Risperdal) has been found to be more effective than other atypical antipsychotics with children diagnosed with ASD who are exhibiting very severe symptoms such as aggression or rage, intense stereotypical and repetitive behavior patterns such as banging of hands or head until they begin to bleed, and severe tantrums and irritability (Julien, 2011). Note that antipsychotics are not prescribed simply because the individual has ASD; they are prescribed only when the individual with ASD exhibits other problematic behaviors as discussed above. However, many researchers warn that these atypical antipsychotics have serious side effects such as weight gain, glucose intolerance, and hyperlipidemia that require the physician to monitor prolactin levels, blood glucose, and body weight (Hollander, Phillips, & Yeh, 2003; Julien et al.). Hollander et al. noted that prescribing atypical antipsychotics at low doses is very effective in improving the hyperactivity and mood instability symptoms exhibited by some individuals with ASD. Although the discussion of medications is best handled by a psychiatrist, it is important that parents educate themselves about the long-term side effects of the psychotropic medications they might be seeking or their children's psychiatrists intend to prescribe.

Some researchers have found a relationship between fatty acid deficiency and the occurrence of ASD (Schuchardt, Huss, Stauss-Grabo, & Hahn, 2010) and have encouraged parents to give their children with ASD Omega 3 supplements (Aman et al., 2009). Although this is an area that needs more extensive research, individuals with ASD who take Omega 3 supplements have not much to lose because the fatty acid supplements produce little or no harm or side effects (Meiri, Bichovsky, & Belmaker, 2009). Overall, the combination of psychotherapy and medication has been found to be most beneficial in cases in which the child with ASD exhibits serious coexisting psychotic symptoms and other problematic and severe behaviors (Julien et al., 2011).

PROBLEMATIC BEHAVIORS AND ASD

The problematic behaviors most commonly seen by educators and parents caring for children or adolescents with ASD in Nigeria are violent behaviors, frequent anger outbursts, impulsivity, and defiance. Inasmuch as violent behavior among school-aged children and teenagers in general is rising in Nigerian society, violent behavior in children and adolescents with ASD could be the result of many factors, some not peculiar to people with ASD. Poor anger management, low tolerance for frustration, and dissatisfaction with the immediate environment may be factors. Violent behaviors observed in children and adolescents with ASD include specific behaviors such as refusing to follow directions or commands from authority figures and verbal aggression, including cursing and disrespect. Monitoring the problematic behaviors of children and adolescents with ASD is very important because of the sometimes unpredictable nature of the violent episodes. Under normal circumstances, predicting violent behavior in a child is relatively easy. But parents, caregivers, and teachers might not see the violent episode coming in a child who exhibits significant communication deficits and lacks social reciprocity.

They also may have difficulty knowing when children with ASD are angry because children with ASD sometimes exhibit neutral (blank) facial expressions. The product of uncontrolled anger is often violent behavior. Uncontrolled and prolonged anger are not only destructive, but they can be deadly as well. Children with ASD might show anger by breaking or destroying objects in their immediate environment, hitting others, fighting, punching the wall or other people, pushing tables or knocking chairs to the floor, and not listening to instructions. Furthermore, although anger is a legitimate emotion and many people express anger at one time or another, parents, teachers, and caregivers need to be familiar with the children with ASD in their sphere of influence to the extent that they are able to detect anger when the children express it and predict the behaviors that are likely to follow. Children who have poor communication and poor motor skills, are impulsive, have serious obsessions, and exhibit very low self-esteem might be difficult to manage when they are angry. Thus, the solution is "catch them before they explode."

UNDERSTANDING DEFIANCE

Basically, defiance is the refusal to follow the directions or the instructions of people in authority such as teachers, principals, parents, older siblings, and caregivers. Defiance is also a trigger to violent acts, and it is indeed violence in and of itself in its broadest sense because it is noncompliance. Some readers may disagree that defiance is violence, so let us explore the meaning of violence. The Merriam Webster Dictionary defines violence as not only physical force, but also as feelings of intensity, profanation, being agitated to the point of experiencing difficulties with self-control, and forceful verbal expressions. Perhaps now readers will agree that defiance is a subset of violence and a child with tendencies toward defiance should not be ignored.

The seriousness of defiance is relative to the environment in which it is displayed. Although parents and educators are encouraged to find ways to curb incidences of defiance that are exhibited by their children with ASD because of the adverse consequences to the children of allowing them to develop defiant patterns of behavior, determining how to handle individual incidences depends on the intensity of the defiant behavior; the intensity will govern whether the behavior is worthy of serious consequences or immediate intervention. For example, if children with ASD are asked to stand up and they initially refuse but later comply, the defiant behavior is not of sufficient intensity to warrant an intervention. On the other hand, if students are asked to stop hitting other students and they continue hitting to the extent that they get into a serious fight, relevant interventions and age appropriate consequences must follow. Students with ASD need to be educated on the need to refrain from violent behaviors such as fighting and they may need to be helped to do so.

Defiance might not necessarily lead to violence but may be indicative of a medical or psychological problem; thus, parents, educators, and caregivers need to exercise good judgment in dealing with defiance. For example, if a child with ASD refuses to eat breakfast after several instructions to do so, if the child throws a tantrum that includes disturbing crying spells, the immediate solution is not always spanking, yelling, or threatening to spank. The immediate reaction should be to investigate the reason for the refusal, especially if the defiance is not the norm for that child. Furthermore, if the child refuses both lunch and dinner as well, the parent should probably take the child to a doctor. The child might be having a medical problem. From the psychological perspective, a child's sudden and persistent refusals to eat are predictors of some affective disorder problems such as depression. For precautionary reasons, know that hunger and thirst are triggers of violent behavior when the defiant behavior is not typical for the child. If, on the other hand, the refusal to eat is typical for the child, it is probably an attention seeking behavior. In that case, parents, caregivers, and teachers are encouraged to implement behavior modification strategies.

UNDERSTANDING VERBAL AGGRESSION

Although it is not common for children with ASD with violent tendencies to exhibit them by being verbally aggressive, it does happen. The verbal aggression might not involve the use of long words that have lots of syllables. Verbal aggression includes cursing, yelling, use of profanities, threats of violence, and the use of verbally abusive language to peers and those in authority. Verbal aggression is most significant when the action is towards an authority figure such as a teacher, caregiver, guardian, or parent. It is of utmost importance for parents, teachers, and caregivers to watch for verbal aggression towards peers as well.

Verbal aggression exhibited by children with ASD is sometimes an imitation of what the children have heard or observed from peers, parents, or neighbors. Thus it is very important to audit the environment to which the child with ASD is exposed. Imitative behaviors are not uncommon amongst the population with ASD. In fact, their mode of learning is often by imitation. What is important to take from this discussion is that violence is also a function of the environment and it can be learned.

PREDICTING VIOLENCE

A number of factors have been associated with violent behavior in the population with ASD as well as in the general population. Common predictors of violence are low self-esteem, fear, mental illness, and certain physical conditions.

Low self-esteem. Quite a lot of discussion has centered on the use of low self-esteem as a predictor of violence in children with ASD. The concept of low self-esteem, which has been viewed as a problem in the western world, is gradually making its way into the Nigerian society. Many Nigerians deny the presence of low self-esteem based on the idea that there is no reason people cannot like themselves. Although low self-esteem has its foundation in dislike of self, feelings of self-pity, and inability to believe in oneself, there is more to low self-esteem than these basics. My definition of low self-esteem as it applies in Nigerian society is the lack of contentment for who one is as a person and confusion about who one wants to be in the future. Many researchers have attempted to discover why people have low self-esteem and also to explore how it can be managed because of its adverse effects on the human person. Although it is beyond the scope of this book to review the research on the many factors and facets of low self-esteem, it is important to know that low self-esteem has been seen to contribute to problem behaviors such as alcoholism, drug addiction, prostitution, suicide, criminality, and other destructive behaviors. Children and adolescents with ASD who exhibit symptoms of low self-esteem are not excluded from such problem behaviors. Violence is indeed one common way that children with ASD show their disapproval for life and other people. This does not mean that all individuals with developmental disabilities have low self-esteem; rather what is relevant here is that children, adolescents, and adults in Nigeria do exhibit low self-esteem despite ignorance of the condition in the society in general. The low self-esteem experienced by children with ASD in Nigeria might stem largely from the stigmatization and the rejection children with ASD frequently face.

Not all children with ASD have obvious physical manifestations of their disorder, and some have average intellectual skills. Thus they ask questions and plan for their future. As they develop into adulthood, they have growing fears that they will neither be accepted for participation in the workforce nor trusted enough to have intimate friendships. The choices that children with ASD make as they advance into adulthood will be productive if they have been appropriately guided and they have a good sense of self. However, without a good sense of self and without a lot of hope, adolescents and adults with ASD might choose lives of crime and violence as a means of survival. In Nigerian society, more work needs to be done to develop activities for the developmentally disabled so their special talents and uniqueness are rewarded from a young age. The persistent belief that individuals with developmental disabilities are incapable of joining the productive workforce is a major hindrance to the creation of opportunities for them. Some philanthropists and church organizations have been dedicated to improving the lives of children, adolescents, and adults in the country with ASD, but more work needs to be done; creating opportunities is the role not only of the government, but also of every citizen of the country of Nigeria. Of course, providing services to children, adolescents, and adults with ASD must begin in the home with the family.

Children with ASD whose families support them in their dreams, weather the dreams are feasible or not, generally have a good sense of self. They feel accepted because they experience the love that is inherent in family cohesiveness. Family cohesiveness helps to validate the love that children experience in their home. In a cohesive family, not merely one person, but all family members are interested in the child. In a cohesive family, children with ASD are treated like their siblings; hence, they don't view themselves as different. Family cohesiveness therefore helps to eradicate fear of rejection in the mind of the individual with ASD. Because children in supportive families usually have good self-esteem and are content with their environment and themselves, they are likely to anticipate an acceptable and eventful future.

To summarize the relationship between self-esteem in children with ASD and violent tendencies: a healthy self-concept breeds peace and contentment with life in general, but low self-esteem can lead to anger, pain, frustration, dissatisfaction, and violence. If a child has nothing to lose or nothing to look forward to in life, why bother? Pleasing and helping a child with ASD with a very low self-concept is difficult because that child has nothing to look forward to in the future to feel happy about. The consequence of an extremely poor concept of self is intense anger. The norm for children with ASD with very low self-concepts is to engage in what I call the "destruction spree." The destruction spree is a series of events that evolves from anger or fear. The spree might first be manifested as general noncompliance and then gradually progresses to verbal aggression and lying behavior, and from there to physical aggression. This destruction spree might also become evident as children with ASD with low self-images respond to changes.

Adapting to change is difficult for most people, and particularly hard for children diagnosed with ASD. Helping children and adolescents with ASD cope with changes requires either some God-given parenting or teaching skills or professional training. Usually, children with ASD resent change, and they show their resentment by crying, seeking attention through any means, or throwing frequent tantrums. Please note that attention seeking behaviors are also products of low self-concept. An attention seeking behavior is simply a cry for attention or an expression of a great need to be approved or accepted by others. When tantrums, crying spells, and attention seeking behaviors do not work, defiance sets in. Consequently, verbal aggression becomes the norm, and verbal aggression gradually becomes physical aggression. It is so important to understand the connection between low self-concept and violence in the child with ASD. Simply stated, low self-concept usually produces discontentment with life and in a discontented life, anger and frustration are the order of the day and the activities of the mind. Built-up anger and frustration lead to gradually increasing displays of violence, outward manifestations of a destruction spree. Though the early violence may not seem out of the ordinary, in time the behaviors become very serious and require significant intervention. Obviously, the best course of action for the child with ASD as well as the people that child affects is to prevent the violence from occurring in the first place. Preventing harm to persons and property is of utmost importance. Prevention of destructive behaviors relies on awareness of the predictors of violence.

Fear. Fear is another factor that impacts violence. You may have heard the expression "fear can kill!" Fear is an emotion that negates love. Fear not only paralyzes the human mind; it also creates stagnation. Fear in children with ASD can exacerbate the symptoms of the disorder; children may refuse to speak or regress in their communication, having increased obsessive behavior patterns, isolate themselves more, and display more repetitive and stereotypical patterns of behavior. Note that the fear experienced by children with ASD might easily be mistaken for psychotic symptom (delusions, hallucinations) or defiance. Fear might be an intrinsic factor of a mental health problem such as depression or anxiety or of a physical problem such as stomach upset, gastroenteritis, or headaches. Uncovering the root of fear in children with ASD is essential to alleviating the fear.

A child with ASD might be afraid of a teacher or a caregiver but exhibit aggression toward peers, parents, or another individual who is not the one causing the fear. This displacement onto an "innocent" target makes identifying the reason for the aggression difficult when it is a result of fear. The problem is compounded by the fact that limitations in communication and intellectual ability often negatively impact reasoning in children with ASD, hampering their understanding of the experiences they encounter on a daily basis. Parents, caregivers, and educators need to be aware that children with ASD who are seriously afraid have no boundaries when it comes to anger and violence. They may react violently toward inanimate objects as well as living creatures. Low functioning individuals with ASD might target violence at any person and at any time.

Other mental illnesses. The presence of depression and anxiety symptoms, such as increased crying spells; reduced appetite or excessive eating; increased or reduced sleep; ongoing nightmares; feelings of worthlessness, hopelessness, or helplessness; increased agitation or anger; and low motivation, can trigger violent behavior. Aggression can result from emotional distress. Coexisting conditions of psychotic disorders such as schizophrenia can trigger violence. In Nigerian society, it is not uncommon to hear bystanders refer to the individuals who are fighting as "crazy" or "mad," parents, caregivers, and teachers must carefully monitor children with ASD with coexisting mental health conditions such as psychosis or depression to prevent incidences of violence or other dangerous behaviors.

Physical problems. Two types of physical problems have been linked to violent tendencies in children with ASD with already existing impulse control difficulties. The first is neurological, manifested in seizures or epilepsy. The most important caution here is that parents, caregivers, and teachers of individuals with autism spectrum disorder diagnosed with seizures or epilepsy should make certain those individuals remain on the medications appropriate for their medical conditions. If you are responsible for a child with ASD who is experiencing frequent seizures, please take that child to a physician for a re-evaluation of medications, for additional brain imaging, for more effective diagnosis, and/or for more assessments to rule out the presence of other medical conditions.

Second, traumatic brain injury (TBI) has also been linked to violent tendencies in children with ASD. Because I have worked in the field of forensic psychology and have conducted comprehensive psychological assessments, I am very concerned about the relationship between TBI and violent behaviors. Without going into detail about the theories and the research that have linked traumatic brain injury to impulsivity and serious violent crimes, let me simply say that the impact of head injuries on emotions can never be overemphasized. Traumatic brain injuries are not always fatal; indeed, some concussions are mild. But injuries to the brain can be very, very serious. Children with

ASD who have serious motor difficulties are always at risk of TBI. Parents and educators must be particularly watchful of their children with ASD when they engage in play, especially if they appear to become out of control with their play. They must monitor the children in the home and outside the home, on the playground and the in classroom, ensuring that children with motor difficulties avoid falls that cause mild or serious injury to the head. The fewer the number of head injuries, the fewer will be the incidents of violent behaviors triggered by TBI.

CASE STUDY: 5-1

Ngozi is a 17-year-old female diagnosed with ASD since age 7. Ngozi has very limited speech and when she hears the voice of a stranger she goes into a closet or the kitchen pantry to avoid being seen. Ngozi is of very small stature and obese. She is not able to feed herself and always seems content. Ngozi is fascinated with her Barbie doll, and the only time she shows any excitement is when she sees a Barbie or someone tries to take the Barbie away from her sight. Ngozi exhibits serious fine motor problems and has difficulties with grasping tightly with either of her hands. Ngozi fidgets a lot and seems fearful when spoken to. Ngozi seldom smiles. Ngozi's parents reported that in the last 9 months, she has been having strange conversations with herself and she is very afraid of darkness.

Her parents stated that sometimes when Ngozi is alone, she moves her lips like she is in a conversation and she smiles at the same time. When asked if she has seen anything, Ngozi responds with a head nod that signifies "yes." Sometimes, Ngozi has had to be redirected back to bed because she tends to sleep walk. Once in a while Ngozi exhibits very scary looks and it seems impossible to understand the reason for the look. Her parents report that recently Ngozi has become scared of water to the extent that she resists taking her bath. The parents report that Ngozi also has imaginary fights, especially at night before she falls asleep. The parents are worried that Ngozi is being tormented at night by evil spirits. The parents fear for the entire family.

On the whole, Ngozi seems to be experiencing a number of problems that fall into the developmental, intellectual, and psychological domains. The fears that her parents are experiencing appear justified. However, their thought that Ngozi might be tormented by evil spirits does not appear rational. In cases similar to that of Ngozi, treatment strategies include the involvement of a psychiatrist, a psychologist, and the special educator. Ngozi will need to be monitored very closely because she is presenting with symptoms of psychosis in addition to the already existing condition of ASD with intellectual disability. In the Nigerian culture, it is not unusual for parents to take children like

Ngozi to a church pastor, an imam, or a traditional healer because they believe evil spirits is involved. Inasmuch as Ngozi's parents might have a strong desire to pursue alleviation of their own fears, their most important responsibility is to seek what is best for Ngozi. From the mental health perspective, Ngozi will show a reduction of symptoms only if her parents cooperate with the treatment regimens suggested by the psychologist and psychiatrist.

The involvement of the teacher is also essential because Ngozi still needs to learn basic life skills. Once the educator is aware of some of Ngozi's presenting symptoms, an individualized education plan that considers those symptoms can be developed for her. Individualized education plans are critical to the life success of children with ASD. Individualized education plans take into consideration not only the educational needs of the student, but also their mental capacity and psychological, physical, and social needs. Parents must encourage their children to follow their individualized education plans because implementation of a carefully developed plan fosters success. A caution: exhibition of strange behaviors by a child with ASD does not necessarily imply schizophrenia. Changes in the child's environment can also trigger unusual behaviors. Parents must not overlook any change that occurs in the life of their child with ASD, and environmental factors have to be ruled out before concluding that any psychosis is present.

CASE STUDY 5-2

Jacob is a 15-year-old male who was diagnosed with ASD at age 4. Jacob resides with his parents and his brother, who is 5 years younger than he. Jacob's parents are both medical doctors and they have sought the best services for Jacob since he was 2 years old. Jacob has received speech therapy since he was 3 years old and he began special school when he was 4. Jacob has a private tutor in the home to help him with his math and he also has a piano teacher. His intellectual abilities are above average and his academic achievements are above average as well. In fact, Jacob and his parents have discussed the possibility of university education. Jacob has also received physical therapy since he was 3 years old because of his extreme motor problems. Although he had problems grasping small objects from a very young age, he has learned how to grasp objects much better as a result of the physical therapy. Jacobs' parents also have a private psychiatrist in the United States who attends to Jacob on a yearly basis. Since the age of 9, Jacob has been taking Risperidone to help with his agitation and extreme restlessness. Recently, Jacob has been exhibiting out-of-control behaviors including hitting his parents and fighting with his brother more frequently. Jacob has been hospitalized and physically restrained in the psychiatric hospital in Nigeria twice this year, and his parents are getting very worried because Jacob is now heavily medicated. Jacob's parents are also worried because they are unable to risk taking Jacob on a long plane trip to the United States for treatment. They are worried that Jacob will become increasingly out of control on the long trip. Although Jacob consistently gained weight since he began taking Risperidone, his weight has doubled since he was placed on the most recent psychotropic medications including Eskalith (Lithium Carbonate), Ativan (Lorazapam), Topamax (Topiramate), Geodon (Ziprasidone), and Cogentin (Benztropine). Jacob was recently diagnosed with diabetes and he is on insulin injections and strong diet control and monitoring. Recently, Jacob has been waking up at night and stealing food from the refrigerator when his parents and brother are asleep. He refuses to attend school and when he is forced to dress for school, he tears his clothes and school uniform and destroys items in his room. His parents are increasingly worried. Jacob, who has always enjoyed his piano lessons, is now resenting his music teacher; he recently punched the music teacher on his back. Jacob's parents are concerned because Jacob is already on several medications, which they think should be able to control his violent tendencies and bizarre behaviors. His parents are also worried because Jacob is extremely overweight and he might beat his brother to the point of death someday. Jacob's parents are seeking help from local psychologists to find the best solution for their son. Although Jacob's parents are seriously considering long term psychiatric treatment or institutionalization for Jacob, they feel guilty for his problems.

Histories of mental illness such as Jacob's are always heartbreaking because the parents have not shown any obvious neglect of the child since he was born. Several hypotheses might explain Jacob's presenting behaviors. From a psychological perspective, there are five major areas of concern:

1. Jacob is a 15-year-old male and, developmentally, he might be experiencing some internal conflicts that might impact his self-esteem.

2. Jacob is currently prescribed lots of psychotropic medications and he is also on insulin injections. The medications may jeopardize Jacob's ability to focus on lessons such as music and math at home. A review of the appropriateness of these medications is warranted even though they were prescribed for his agitation and aggression, which are still intense. Sometimes reducing or discontinuing these medications result in significant changes. But the effects of different dosages of different medications vary with each patient; it is the role of the psychiatrist to review the medications and prescribe a new regimen if appropriate.

3. Jacob is significantly overweight. This fact, coupled with the fact Jacob is in puberty, indicates a need to review his diet closely as well as the diets of all the family members. Jacob probably does not want to be the only one in the house deprived of foods he deems tasty.

4. Jacob might be resisting going to school because he feels he does not belong or because he is being bullied or teased. Thus, he is afraid! Does Jacob have friends at school? Not having friends at school would intensify the feeling that he doesn't belong. Another reason Jacob resists attending school could be attributed to his need to sleep more. The high number of psychotropic medications can affect sleep, and the fact that he wakes up at night to steal food from the refrigerator suggests he might not be getting enough rest at night. Both lack of rest and hunger are possible triggers of violent behaviors.

5. Jacob has been diagnosed with diabetes mellitus. This condition does not make life easy for either Jacob or his parents. In the Nigerian culture, this situation would be called "double wahala," or in English, a "double problem." However, it is not the end of the world for Jacob and his family. His diabetes can be effectively controlled with diet, exercise, and medications. The question then is: How active is Jacob? Is he on any physical activity or exercise regimen? The presence of the parents is most important at this critical time of Jacob's life. It is not enough to have a loving nanny and an intelligent tutor for Jacob.

In conclusion, the case study of Jacob (5-2) illustrates the complex nature of the behaviors of children and adolescents with ASD. The development of an effective treatment plan and provision of the best services for children diagnosed with ASD are the responsibility of the children's parents, and that responsibility does not end if the children have all the resources available to help them achieve their dreams. Developmental conditions such as puberty, medical problems such as diabetes mellitus, emotional problems such as aggression and impulsivity, and environmental factors in the home and the school are not static. Parents, caregivers, and educators need to continually evaluate the types of services their children with ASD receive at each stage of their development. Monitoring the children and observing new behaviors is the role of the parent more than of the educator or the sibling. Most importantly, the power of "presence" in the life of the child with ASD cannot be emphasized enough. The "presence" children with ASD living in Nigeria desire will always exceed the care the children receive from a paid nanny or baby sitter. The precious presence of loving parents is greater than any gift of toys or amenities the child will ever receive. Presence has to do with quality, not merely quantity.

PART TWO
TIPS FOR MANAGING PROBLEM BEHAVIORS

This second part of *Autism Spectrum Disorder: A Guide for Educators and Parents* provide tried and true ideas for managing problem behaviors of individuals diagnosed with an ASD. Some teachers have five or more students with ASD in their classrooms at one time, and helping all of them develop the skills they need while controlling their difficult behaviors is an enormous challenge. Parents also have many ongoing challenges in helping their children with ASD. Other teachers and parents as well as many researchers have found interventions and strategies that have worked with individuals with ASD with problem behaviors. Some of these are offered here as tips for parents, caregivers, and teachers to explore in their own situations.

REVIEW OF PROBLEM BEHAVIORS

For individuals with autism spectrum disorder, managing behavior becomes complicated when multiple etiologies accompany the condition. Medical and neurological problems compound behavior challenges; seizures, gastroenteritis, slurred speech, difficulty holding or grasping objects, fine motor skills difficulty, obesity, difficulty maintaining balance, diabetes mellitus, and many more possible medical and neurological problems make everyday activities hard for individuals with ASD. Psychological problems, which include depression, psychosis or schizophrenia, anxiety, high stress, low self-esteem, attention deficit hyperactivity disorder, obsessive compulsive disorder, as well as others, impact behavior. The major behavior problems parents and teachers struggle with in individuals with ASD are defiance, aggression, poor anger control, low frustration tolerance, and crying spells.

FOUNDATIONS FOR MANAGING THE CHALLENGING BEHAVIORS

The foundations for successful management of the challenging behaviors exhibited by individuals with ASD are accurate diagnosis, structure and consistency, communication, psychiatric medications, and nutritional foods.

Diagnosis. Diagnosing ASD and identifying challenging behaviors is a three-step process. First, a clinical psychologist interviews parents, caregivers, and teachers for a preliminary assessment. Second, the psychologist administers multiple batteries of specific psychological tests to confirm the presence of ASD symptoms and identify the behaviors specific to the individual. ASD is a spectrum disorder, which means that different individuals with ASD present with different behaviors. Third, after the psychological assessment is completed, the psychologist talks further with the child or adult's parents, caregivers, and teachers and together they develop a treatment plan. Note that the discussion here does not address using diagnostic results for appropriate class placements; this is a very broad topic that will be examined at length in a future publication.

Without digressing too far, let me observe that misdiagnosis is on the rise and the adverse effects of misdiagnosis are serious.

Thus, I state that diagnosis is just as important as treatment or intervention. As you must know, you cannot cure what you don't know you have. To the many parents or caregivers who resist professional diagnosis because of their different belief systems or religious inclinations, it is necessary to add that "Faith" in a supreme being or a higher power entails using all the resources available that increases knowledge, provide understanding, and enhance healing. Remember, human beings are involved—their wellbeing and their future—so obtaining an accurate diagnosis is extremely important.

Structure and consistency. Although I cannot stress enough the importance of structure and consistency for the individual with ASD, permit me to explain what structure means for the individual with ASD. Structure entails consistency in implementing any plans and in organizing day to day activities. Structure prevents the individual with ASD from being confronted with too many preventable surprises. The number of new things that individuals with ASD can tolerate depends on their mental health functioning and level of impairment. Please note that structure means consistency, not rigidity. Rigidity is not only negative, but also has the impact of impeding the social development of the individual diagnosed with ASD. Consistency enables the individual to practice social skills through repetition.

Communication. Structure requires that people communicate effectively. That is, those in authority speak *with* individuals with ASD rather than speak *at* them because of their impairment. Words spoken in an authoritative, threatening, and formal manner are far different from words delivered in a non-threatening, friendly, and informal way. As you know, individuals with ASD are extremely sensitive to threats. Effective communication allows the person in authority (teacher, administrator, parent, caregiver, older sibling, etc.) not only to observe the times and triggers of problem behaviors, but also to teach positive replacement behaviors appropriately. Positive replacement behaviors are taught by modeling good behavior, role playing good behavior, telling stories to promote acceptable behavior, and directly teaching acceptable social skills. Integrating humor with the teaching of replacement behaviors can sometimes be effective because humor reduces feelings of stress and nervousness. Please note that the use of humor must be controlled so the reason for the communication is not lost.

Psychiatric medications. Sometimes, depending on the severity of the physical symptoms exhibited by the individual with ASD and the presence of any co-morbid mental health disorders (depression, psychosis, anxiety, etc.), psychiatric medications might be prescribed. Care must be taken not to overmedicate the individual with ASD. The long-term adverse effects of excessive psychotropic medications are not pleasant. Seeking the opinion of a psychiatrist is of utmost importance. At times, parents or caregivers might need to seek the opinions of more than one psychiatrist; obtaining more than one recommendation is strongly encouraged if parents are in doubt or are not convinced of the wisdom of the decision to medicate. If any doubt exists, by all means take the individual with ASD to see more than one psychiatrist. Additionally, learn what side effects to expect from the medications the individual with ASD is taking so you can report any symptoms that concern you to the treating psychiatrist in a timely manner.

Nutrition. The need for nutritional foods cannot be over-emphasized because of the positive benefits healthy eating has on the individual with ASD. Foods rich in amino acids and low in sugar are very effective for keeping the challenging behaviors of individuals with ASD in check.

A MODEL FOR MANAGING CHALLENGING BEHAVIORS

I have developed a model that has been very helpful for ongoing behavior management for developmentally disabled children or adults exhibiting serious behavior problems. As you know, autism spectrum disorder is classified as a developmental disability. The model is built on solid principles of cognitive-behavioral theory, behavior theory, reality theory, and systems theory. Rather than bore you with psychological jargon by explaining the various counseling theories, let me simply describe the model. I call it the BAASIC model; BAASIC is an acronym for its six components:

B - Behavior
A - Antecedents
A - Action
S - Succedents
I - Interventions
C - Change

You may ask, "What is an antecedent? And what on earth does succedents mean?" Mathematicians and statisticians are familiar

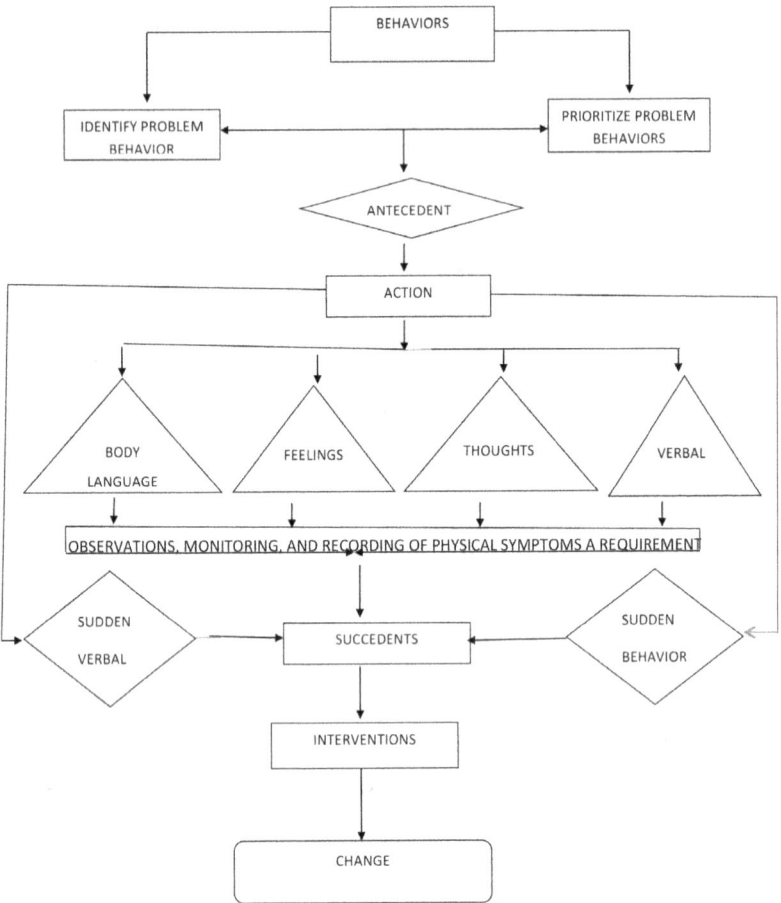

with the terms antecedent and succedent. Although logicians have complicated definitions, they are not difficult to understand.
Figure 1. BAASIC model of behavior management for pervasive developmental disorder.

Basically, antecedents and succedents are phenomena that can be observed. In the BAASIC model, antecedents and succedents are observable truths. These observable truths form the framework for the behavior change that parents, teachers, or caregivers desire. The prefix "ante" means before, and antecedents come before behavior; antecedents are the triggers for the problem behavior. The prefix "succeed" means after and succedents come after the behavior; they are the gains the individual receives from the problem behavior. Accurately identifying the antecedents and succedents increases the chance of changing the problem behavior. Note that although the behavior is problematic, the antecedents and succedents are not necessarily negative.

Utilizing the BAASIC model enables the parent, teacher, or therapist to address the problem behavior with the goal of teaching appropriate ways of responding to the antecedents and achieving the succedents. Note however, that changing a behavior is like solving a puzzle. The process can be frustrating until the desired result is achieved. Once the puzzle is solved, the feelings of relief and relaxation are far greater than the anxiety that was felt when the puzzle was not solved. So do not be discouraged when you experience resistance as you attempt to help individuals change problematic and challenging behaviors. Keep trying and remember that changing the problem behavior is the goal. Keep your focus on the problem behavior and attempt to separate the human beings from the behaviors they exhibit. Allow me now to go through the BAASIC model and show how to use it as an instrument for changing challenging behaviors.

Step 1. *Identify the problem behavior* - Most times, the individual with ASD has more than one problem behavior. Write down the problem behaviors you observe. Once you have a list, prioritize the problem behaviors, ranking them in order of which behavior is most disturbing and needs immediate attention. Prioritize according to how frequently the behavior occurs and how it impacts the health and safety not only of the individual, but also of others around the individual.

Step 2. *Identify the antecedents* - It is important that you identify the antecedents for each problem behavior. To reiterate, antecedents are the factors that trigger the behavior to occur. Assumptions are not antecedents. There is always a trigger, sometimes visible and sometimes invisible.

Step 3. *Identify the action behaviors* - Action behaviors are the problem or challenging behaviors that are easily observed. Action behaviors are different from the behaviors in Step 1. The problem behavior in Step 1 is the end behavior observed (such as hitting a classmate); action behaviors are the first signals that the individual is upset or unhappy (such as waving hands rapidly). Identifying the action behaviors that precede the problem behavior is important. Sometimes, the antecedents are confused for the action behavior. A classmate taking a toy is an antecedent; the child with ASD hopping from one foot to the other in response is an action behavior; the student pushing the classmate is the problem behavior. Note that it is only after you have identified the action behaviors that you will be able to address the antecedents and then the problem behavior. The guidelines for identifying the action behaviors are as follows:

a. What body language is easily observable?
b. What feelings are exhibited to suggest that a problem behavior has been triggered?
c. What thoughts do you perceive preceded the feelings?
d. Is the action behavior sudden, unpredictable, and non-verbal? Or is the action behavior sudden, unpredictable, and verbal or physical?
e. What indeed is the action behavior?

Step 4. *Identify the succedents* - The succedents are the benefits of the problem behavior for the individual with ASD. Succedents are not necessarily negative. Basically, what does the individual gain from the behavior? This can be extremely difficult to determine, especially when parents, teachers, or caregivers allow their emotion to get in the way of objectivity. Let us remember that the cognitive or intellectual abilities of the student with ASD might not be sophisticated. However, I do not want to minimize the frustrations that some of their problem behaviors cause parents and teachers. The goal is to find a solution to the problem. My suggestion, therefore, is to remain solution focused. Once our goal is to find solutions to the difficult problem behavior, we are up for success. Please do not get discouraged with some of your objective findings about the gratification enjoyed by the student with ASD from any of the problem behaviors. Individuals with ASD are teachable, and they can change if we approach them with love and empathy. The goal is to teach them how to achieve the positive succedents they want without the challenging behaviors.

Step 5. *Identify the interventions-* Interventions address the problem behavior, which is encircled by antecedents and suc-cedents. Behavioral counselors refer to a variety of principles in different counseling theories in selecting interventions, but I will keep suggestions for interventions rather simple. Keeping in mind that the individuals involved are developmentally challenged, you should apply the following rules to choosing interventions. The interventions must:

a.   Be age appropriate

b.   Be structured and monitored

c.   Fit the problem behavior

d.   Include positive antecedents and succedents

e.   Be consistent

f.   Be measurable so success can be determined

g.   Be completed in a specified time

h.   Be administered in simple and clear language

The interventions may be time outs, rewarding positive behaviors and providing consequences for negative behaviors, and education. Time outs can be very effective for individuals who function developmentally within the age range of 1-6 years. However, time outs and other punitive interventions (e.g., spanking) can be very detrimental to the self-esteem of the children with ASD. Thus, my advice is to be cautious.

I am a great advocate for using education, which I call "talking the behavior," to effect change. What does this mean? The individual with ASD is invited to have a conversation to discuss the problem behavior. Note that the word "conversation" is positive; it does not set the individual apart. When I was a school teacher, students with negative behaviors quickly opted to choose good behaviors during class times because they did not want to be in a long conversation with me. Not many of the students enjoyed conversations with me when the conversations were about my agenda. On the other hand, if a conversation is based on the students' agenda, the students and probably the teacher as well are interested and the conversation is therefore more productive. Some of the interesting conversations we had were about how the students displayed good behaviors throughout the day, how I needed to reward them for their positive behaviors, and their positive attitudes toward class work.

Confronting an individual who is developmentally delayed can be quite an effective intervention, but it must be done in a non-threatening manner. When individuals with ASD are confronted with their triggers and their succedents, their initial reaction is usually silence. After the confrontation, you can discuss how detrimental the negative behavior is to them, their family members, and other people who might be living with them.

Another intervention is ignoring the problem behavior. When one of the succedents is attention, ignoring the behavior can be effective. But note that ignoring is a means to changing the behavior and not the end of the targeted problem behavior. Always remember that low or poor self-esteem is an issue for individuals with ASD and is often the reason for attention-seeking behaviors. To reduce the problem behaviors, individuals with ASD need to be taught positive ways of gaining attention once the ignoring message is communicated and allowed to take effect.

Behaviorist, parents, and teachers have used rewards and consequences for many years as both a means and an end in changing problem behaviors. They reward positive behaviors, possibly providing antecedents, by giving tokens of some sort. Rewards are not necessarily money or expensive gifts. Rewards can be verbal praise, complements, watching television, playing longer hours before taking showers, singing favorite songs, drawing, and other activities. Consequences could be not watching a favorite television program or not playing with favorite toys or games. The key with implementing the rewards and consequences strategy is to be sure that the individual understands the reason for the reward or the consequence. The strategy is an ineffective intervention if the individual does not recognize that receiving the reward or the consequence is the result of exhibiting specific behaviors. In the BAASIC model, the goal is to prevent the problem behaviors. Use of rewards and consequences can remove the triggers for the behaviors (antecedents). The intervention also addresses succedents because it rewards appropriate ways of seeking attention, thus preventing tantrums.

Other interventions include training in anger management; moral education; and seeking the help of a psychiatrist, a physical therapist, a nutritionist, or a psychologist. Choosing the right intervention for the particular problem behavior is the key to long lasting positive change. The focus of the intervention phase is to teach the individual with ASD positive ways to prevent the antecedents and also enjoy the succedents they truly desire.

Step 6. *Identify the behavior change* - At this stage, if the first five steps have been implemented properly, some changes will occur. In individuals with ASD, change comes in fragments. Let us applaud and validate the changes when they occur, no matter how small. Regardless of how minute the change is, a positive change is a good thing, and even a smile from the parent, teacher, or caregiver is validation. Just as a river is formed from little drops of water, positive behavior is developed in stages, from small validations and ongoing teaching of appropriate ways of behaving.

CASE SCENARIO

Jonah is a 9-year-old male with ASD who recently began crying excessively about everything, including when he is being fed or bathed. Jonah is being raised by his mother, who is extremely frustrated with his behavior, and she is seeking help from Jonah's class teacher on how to manage his behavior. The teacher recommended that Jonah's mother be more firm with him and characterized Jonah as manipulative and a "spoiled child." The mother said she had ongoing struggles getting Jonah to eat meals daily. She stated that she gives him vitamins to make him feel hungry, but Jonah continues to refuse his meals and resists bathing. In addition to ASD, he has been diagnosed with intellectual disability and has problems with his fine motor skills. Jonah is not able to hold any object with either hand. Jonah is taking multiple psychotropic medications to stabilize his mood but he continues to cry a lot. The class teacher is frustrated because Jonah has not attended school consistently. The class teacher requests better attendance, but Jonah's mother stated that he refuses to go to school. Sometimes, because she is fed up with the situation, his mother allows Jonah to get his way, permitting him to not go to school or not take his shower or bath. The mother's perception that the teacher does not understand the intensity of her problems frustrates her considerably, and she feels alone and helpless.

How do we help Jonah using the BAASIC model?

Step 1. *Identify the problem behavior.* Jonah has at least three problem behaviors: increased crying spells, refusing food and shower/bathing, and refusing to go to school. We prioritize them in the following order: (1) refusing food and shower/bathing, (2) crying spells, (3) refusing to go to school.

You will notice that top priority goes to bath and food. This is because these are activities that are essential for survival. Without food and appropriate hygiene, medical complications which could be detrimental to the child's health and also to the health of others who interact closely with the child could occur. I know you might think that school should be more important. But a child who refuses to eat or take a bath cannot function well in school. How can a child who does not eat focus in school? Will anyone want to sit close to a child who has not had a bath or shower for more than 1 or 2 days? Not necessarily! The psychological implications of neglect of personal hygiene are enormous, including low self-esteem; increased isolation, which is not good for children or adolescents with ASD with already poor social interaction skills; and depression. Sometimes individuals with ASD who are on medications for psychiatric conditions experience physical side effects such as increased weight and drooling. You want those children or adults to have appropriate hygiene practices. Furthermore, crying spells, if allowed to continue, will also impact school negatively. Thus, this behavior is ranked as second and school attendance is ranked third.

Step 2. *Identify the antecedents.* What are the triggers for Jonah's behaviors? The parent or caregiver is in the best position to identify the true triggers for Jonah's behavior. Based on the limited information we have, these questions can guide us to identify the antecedents:

a. Does he have any medical or psychiatric problems?

b. Has the structure of activities in the house changed?

c. Is Jonah waking up earlier now than in the past?

d. Does Jonah have unresolved anger management problems?

e. Is Jonah experiencing more communication difficulties?

f. Has Jonah begun new medications that might have side effects?

g. Is Jonah having nightmares or other difficulty sleeping?

h. Are the parents experiencing financial difficulties or have Jonah's meals changed?

For the purpose of illustration, we will say the antecedent for Jonah's refusing to shower is identified as rashes on his skin and the antecedent for his crying spells is increased attention seeking. The antecedent for not going to school is identified as fear.

Step 3. *Identify the action behaviors.* Jonah's major actions are feelings and thoughts of disapproval and body language that suggests some pain or anger. His actions are non-verbal and predictable. Identifying the actions is quite easy here because the problem behaviors are linked to specific observable activities—namely, not taking baths or showers, not eating, and refusing to go to school. To be more specific, Jonah's action behaviors relating to not bathing are refusing to enter the bathroom and refusing to take off his clothes. The action behaviors related to the crying spells are refusing to speak or respond to questions, increased odd behaviors, and exhibiting sad looks. Related to not going to school, the action behaviors are refusing to put on school clothes and resisting coming out of the home.

Step 4. *Identify the succedents.* The benefit of refusing to shower for Jonah is reduced pain when water is poured on his skin, and the benefits of the crying spells are increased attention, being allowed to tell his favorite story, being allowed to watch television, and being given a cup of orange juice. One benefit of refusing school might be avoiding confrontations from peers or teachers that trigger fear. Please note that the succedents, or gains from negative behaviors, might be intrinsic or extrinsic. Succedents can also be positive or negative. An example of a negative gain is acting-out behavior that promotes laziness; an example of a positive gain is increased attention. Without gain, there would be no acting-out behavior. By the same token, because the same gains can be achieved through behaviors that are not problematic, interventions can be implemented that effect positive change.

Step 5. *Identify the interventions.* The actual interventions are dependent on the problem behaviors, action behaviors, antecedents, and succedents. Let us now focus on Jonah's refusal to take baths or showers. The intervention requires finding alternatives to showering or taking baths. Although the alternatives might not have the same effect as actually taking a bath or shower, consideration of the antecedents and the succedents are necessary to eradicate the problem behavior. Let us be honest: sometimes parents create more problems for themselves because of their ardent desire to provide the best for their children. The best might be what makes the child uncomfortable. Jonah is requesting to be freed from pain. One intervention for his excessive crying might be teaching him how to request to spend more time watching television or narrating his favorite stories. Other appropriate interventions for Jonah could also be time outs, rewards and consequences. Jonah can be rewarded when he appropriately verbalizes his needs (antecedents) and the consequence of not being allowed to view his favorite program on television (succedent) can be applied when crying spells continue. Notice, identifying and using the antecedents and the succedents are very important to changing any negative behavior.

Step 6. *Identify the behavior change.* After implementing the intervention, we expect that change will take place. If it does not, go back to Step 1 and address the identified behaviors again. Perhaps you overlooked or misread some antecedents, succedents, and action behaviors. Change is the ultimate goal of the BAASIC model. Be patient, observant, and persistent. The effort it takes to go through the steps of the model will pay off in time.

REFERENCES

American Psychiatric Association. (2000). *Diagnostic and statistical manual of mental disorders – Test Revision* (4th ed. rev.). Washington DC: Author.

Adewuya, A. O., & Famuyiwa, O. O. (2007). Attention deficit hyperactivity disorder among Nigerian primary school children: Prevalence and co-morbid conditions. *European Child Adolescent Psychiatry, 16,* 10-15.

Ajuwon, P. M., & Brown, I. (2012). Family quality of life in Nigeria. *Journal of Intellectual Disability Research, 56* (1), 61-70.

Aman, M. G., McDougle, C. J., Scahill, L., Handen, B., Arnold, L. E., Johnson, C., . . . Stigler, K. (2009). Medication and parent training in children with pervasive developmental disorders and serious behavioral problems: Results from a randomized clinical trial. *Journal of the American Association of Child and Adolescent Psychiatry, 48,* 1143-1154.

Attwood, T. (2008). *The complete guide to Asperger's syndrome.* Philadelphia: Jessica Kingsley Publishers.

Bakare, M. O., Ebigbo, P. O., & Ubochi, V. N. (2012). Prevalence of autism spectrum disorder among Nigerian children with intellectual disability: A stopgap assessment. *Journal of*

Health Care for the Poor and Underserved, 23 (2), 513-518. doi:10.1353/hpu.2012.0056

Barnes, K. A., Howard, J. H., Jr., Howard, D. V., Gilotty, L., Kenworthy, L., Gaillard, W. D., & Vaidya, C. J. (2008). Intact implicit learning of spatial context and temporal sequences in childhood autism spectrum disorder. *Neuropsychology, 22* (5), 563-570.

Desoto, M. C., & Hitlan, R. T. (2007). Blood levels of mercury are related to diagnosis of autism: A reanalysis of an important data set. *Journal of Neurology, 22*, 1308-1311.

Ebesutani, C., Reise, S. P., Chorpita, B. F., Ale, C., Regan, J., Young, J., . . . Weisz, J. R. (2012). The revised child anxiety and depression scale – short version: Scale reduction via exploratory bifactor modeling of the broad anxiety factor. *Psychological Assessment, 24* (4), 833-845.

Egbikuadje, A. A. (2005). The psychosocial and cultural variables affecting adolescents living with parent(s) infected with the AIDS virus in selected states of the Niger Delta region of Nigeria. Fresno, CA: Alliant International University.

Estes, A., Rivera, V., Bryan, P.C., & Dawson, G. (2011). Discrepancies between academic achievement and intellectual ability in higher-functioning school-aged children with autism spectrum disorder. *Journal of Autism and Developmental Disorders, 41*, 1044-1052.

Feldman, R. S. (2003). *Development across the life span* (3rd ed.). Upper Saddle River, NJ: Prentice Hall.

Gadow, K. D., DeVincent, C. J., & Pomeroy, J. (2006). ADHD symptoms subtypes in children with pervasive developmental disorder. *Journal of Autism and Developmental Disorders, 36,* 271-283.

Gjevik, E., Eldevik, S., Fjaeran-Granum, T., & Sponheim, E. (2011). Kiddie-SADS reveals high rates of DSM-IV disorders in children and adolescents with autism spectrum disorders. *Journal of Autism and Developmental Disorders, 41,* 761-769.

Guttmann-Steinmetz, S., Gadow, K. D., DeVincent, C. J., & Crowell, J. (2010). Anxiety symptoms in boys with autism spectrum disorder, attention-deficit hyperactivity disorder, or chronic multiple tic disorder and community controls. *Journal of Autism and Developmental Disorders, 40,* 1006-1016.

Hollander, E., Phillips, A., & Yeh, C. (2003). Targeted treatments for symptoms domains in child and adolescent autism. *Lancet, 362* (9385), 732-734.

Hillier, A. J., Fish, T., Siegel, J. H., & Beversdorf, D. Q. (2011). Social and vocational skills training reduces self-reported anxiety and depression among young adults on the autism spectrum. *Journal of Developmental and Physical Disabilities, 3,* 267-276.

Igbinovia, J. (2012, November 18). Reasons for misdiagnosis of autism in Nigeria. *Vista Woman.* Retrieved from www.vanguardngr.com

Jones, C. R. G., Happe, F., Golden, H., Marsden, A. J. S., Tregay, J., Simonoff, E., . . . Charman, T. (2009). Reading and arithmetic in adolescents with autism spectrum disorders: Peaks and dips in attainment. *Neuropsychology, 23,* 718-728.

Julien, R. M., Advokat, C. D., & Comaty, J. E. (2011). *A primer of drug action: A comprehensive guide to the actions, uses, and side effects of psychoactive drugs* (12th ed.). New York: Worth Publishers.

Kolvin, I. (1972). Emotional problems of childhood and adolescence-Infantile autism or infantile psychosis. *British Medical Journal, 3,* 753-755.

Kuhlthau, K., Orlich, F., Hall, T. A., Sikora, D., Kovacs, E. A., Delahaye, J., & Clemons, T. E. (2010). Health-related quality of life in children with autism spectrum disorders: Results from the autism treatment network. *Journal of Autism and Developmental Disorders, 40,* 721-729. doi:10.1007/s10803-009-0921-2

Leekam, S. R., Prior, M. R., & Uljarevic, M. (2011). Restricted and repetitive behaviors in autism spectrum disorders: A review of research in the last decade. *Psychological Bulletin, 137,* 562-593.

Linn, M. C., & Peterson, A. C. (1985). Emergence and characterization of sex difference in spatial ability: A meta analysis. *Child Development, 56,* 1479-1498.

Luyster, R., & Lord, C. (2009). Word learning in children with autism spectrum disorders. *Developmental Psychology, 45,* 1774-1786.

Matson, J. L., & Sturmey, P. (2011). *International handbook of autism and pervasive developmental disorders.* New York: Springer.

McAlonan, G. M., Suckling, J., Wong, N., Cheung, V., Lienenkaemper, N., Cheung, C., & Chua, S. E. (2008). Distinct patterns of grey matter abnormality in high functioning autism and Asperger's syndrome. *Journal of Child Psychology and Psychiatry, 49*, 1287-1295.

Meiri, G., Bichovsky, Y., & Belmaker, R. (2009). Omega-3 fatty acid treatment in autism. *Journal of Child and Adolescent Psychopharmacology, 19*, 449-451.

Minuchin, S. (1974). *Families and family therapy*. Cambridge, MA: Harvard University Press. In R. H. Mikessell, D.-D. Lusterman, & S. H. McDaniel (Eds., 2001) *Integrating family therapy: Handbook of family psychology and systems theory* (p. 117). Washington DC: American Psychological Association.

Muris, P., & Meesters, C. (2002). Symptoms of anxiety disorders and teacher-reported school functioning of normal children. *Psychological Reports, 91*, 588-590.

Nwokolo, O. M. (2010). A psychologist's perspective on the taboo of autism in Nigeria. Retrieved from www.autism aroundtheglobe.org/countries/Nigeria.asp

Possey, D. J., & McDougle, C. J. (2008). The pharmacology of target symptoms associated with autistic disorder and other pervasive developmental disorders. *Harvard Review of Psychiatry, 8*(2), 45-63.

Sattler, J. M. (2001). *Assessment of children cognitive applications* (4rd ed.). San Diego, CA: Jerome M. Sattler Publisher, Inc.

Schuchardt, J. P., Huss, M., Stauss-Grabo, M., & Hahn, A. (2010). Significance of long-chain-polyunsaturated fatty acids (PUFAs) for the development and behavior of children. *European Journal of Pediatrics, 169*, 149-164.

Strain, P. S., Schwartz, I. S., & Barton, E. E. (2011). Providing interventions for young children with autism spectrum disorders. *Journal of Early Intervention, 33*, 321-332.

Strang, J., F., Kenworthy, L., Daniolos, P., Case, L., Wills, M. C., Martin, A., & Wallace, G. (2012). Depression and anxiety symptoms in children and adolescents with autism spectrum disorders without intellectual disability. *Research in autism spectrum disorders, 6* (1) 406-412.

Sugranyes, G., Kyriakopoulos, M., Corrigall, R., Taylor, E., & Frangou, S. (2011). Autism spectrum disorders and schizophrenia: Meta-analysis of the neural correlates of social cognition. *PLoS One, 6*(10), e25322. doi:10.1371/journal.pone.0025322

Toal, F., Bloemen, O. J., Deeley, Q., Tunstall, N., Daly, E. M., Page, L., . . . Murphy, D. G. M. (2009). Psychosis and autism: Magnetic resonance imaging study of brain anatomy. *British Journal of Psychiatry, 194*, 418-425. doi: 10.1192/bjp.bp.107.049007

Young, G. S., Rogers, S. J., Hutman, T., Rozga, A., Sigman, M., & Ozonoff, S. (2011). *Developmental Psychology. 47*, 1565-1578.

SUBJECT INDEX

A

Academic Performance
  (see intelligence)
Adaptive Functioning, 35

Affective Disorders, 16, 61, 91
Aggression, 67, 89-99
Antecedents (See BAASIC model)
Anxiety, 15, 61-66, 70-74
Attention Deficit Hyperactivity
  Disorder (ADHD), 38-42
Awareness, 37-59

B

BAASIC Model, 111-123

Boundaries, 30, 43, 56,
  72, 97

C

Causes of "ASDs," 17

Challenging Behaviors, 108-118

Communications, 4, 26-29, 109

D

Defiance, 45, 51, 56-57,
  88-91, 96
Depression, 62-70, 73, 77,
  91, 97-98, 107
Developmental Mile-
  stones, 7-8, 12-13
Distractibility (See ADHD)

www.ingramcontent.com/pod-product-compliance
Lightning Source LLC
Chambersburg PA
CBHW060902280326
41934CB00007B/1152